FORENSIC WELLNESS® WORKBOOK

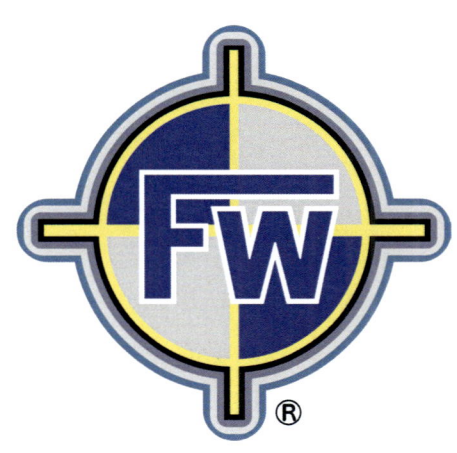

A Workbook and Companion to Forensic Wellness® by

ROBERT McELROY, Ph.D.

Forensic Wellness® Workbook
A Workbook and Companion to *Forensic Wellness®*
Copyright © 2023 by Robert C. McElroy, Ph.D. All rights reserved.

No part of this book may be reproduced or transmitted in any written, electronic, recording, or photocopying form or by any means without written permission from the author. The exception would be in the case of brief quotations where permission is specifically granted by the publisher or author.

Author's Material Content Organization: Carolyn Sorrell
Editors: Dawn Lee Wakefield and Agnes McElroy
Cover and Logo Design: Robert McElroy

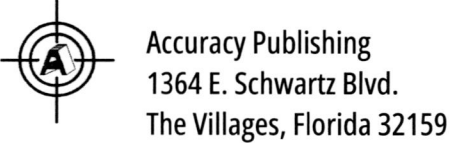

Accuracy Publishing
1364 E. Schwartz Blvd.
The Villages, Florida 32159

ISBN trade softcover: 978-1-7370849-2-1

First Edition
Printed in the USA

10 9 8 7 6 5 4 3 2 1

Contents

Highway 1: Why Highways Instead of Chapters? 2
    Go Forward Proactively—Your Highway To Wellness 2

Highway 2: Forensic STEM Wellness & Weight Loss = Train Your Mind to Lose Weight Permanently ... 4
    How Do I Do This? 4
    Change Your Story—Change Your Lifestyle 4
    How Do I See Myself? 4
    ACT! 6

Highway 3: Let's Get Started! What is Wellness Visioning? 8
    Key Terms 8
    Three Foundational Steps: 8
    What is the MIND Diet? 8
    Vision and Implementation 8

Highway 4: Your Challenges Today 12
    Facts About Obesity 12
    Do you fall into this category? 12

Highway 5: Weight Tracking and Food Measurement Scales 14

Highway 6: Challenges and A Plan 16
    Spectator or Participant? 16
    A regular eating plan is the best solution to overeating.. 18

Highway 7: What Does STEM Mean? 20
    STEM stands for: 20

Highway 8: Realistic Weight Control 22
    STEM To Lose Weight 22
    Mathematically Calculating Weight Loss 22
    Your Plan for Weight Control 24
    How the STEM Plan Can Help 24

Highway 9: Critical Chain to Success 26
    How to Arrive at the Number of Calories Your Body Requires Each Day 26

Highway 10: Your Specific Goals 28
    Cognitive Behavioral Therapy (CBT) 28

Highway 11: Selected Diets Backed by Science 30
    Guidelines for the MIND diet 30

Highway 12: Think Globally but Act Locally and Personally 32

Highway 13: Your Personal Weigh-In 34
    Your Scale and Tracking System 34

Highway 14: Key Steps to Successful Weight Loss 38
    Let's begin by asking ourselves 4 important questions: 38

Highway 15: Question #1—Why Are You Overweight? 40

Highway 16: Question #2—Can I Lose Weight in a Healthy Manner? 42
    Some Reasons Why You Might Overeat? 42

Highway 17: Maintaining target weight: How family and friends may affect your journey ... 44

Highway 18: Sustaining Your Physique 46

Highway 19: STEM Plan Reality vs. Self-Delusion 48

Highway 20: A Sustainable Weight Loss Plan 50

Highway 21: The Real You 52

Highway 22: Healthy Food Costs 54

Highway 23: Take Suggestions and Make Decisions 56

Highway 24: Is Achieving Your Weight Loss the Equivalent of the Moon Shot? 58

Highway 25: Dieting Is Not as Far as Away as the Moon 60
    How Difficult Is It to Lose Weight? 60

Highway 26: Lose and Maintain Your Desired Weight 62

Highway 27: Set a Target! 64

Highway 28: Determine the Right Calorie Number 64

Highway 29: For Women Only 66

Highway 30: For Women & Men 68

Highway 31: Commitment 70

Highway 32: Equilibrium Value 72
    You will develop new and more healthy relationships with food. 72

Highway 33: Critical Mass (CM) and Equilibrium Value (EV) 74

Highway 34: WLC, WLM, and Bounce 74

Highway 35: Stay on the Highway. Don't Exit to a Sideroad 76

Highway 36: Meal Planning 76

Highway 37: One-Day Calorie Count 78

Highway 38: Realistic Weight Loss Expectation & Plan 78

Highway 39: Personal Checklist 80

    You Can Lose Weight 80

    Personal and Honest Reality Check. 80

    Go-To Foods 80

    Foods to Avoid Include:. 80

Highway 40: Math—Daily, Monthly, and Yearly Weight Loss. 82

Highway 41: Math Utilization Areas. 84

    Weight Loss Tools 84

    Identify Potential "Slippery Slopes" 84

    Proactive Decision Making 84

    Healthy Weight and Body. 84

Highway 42: Social and Peer Pressure 86

Highway 43: Target Weight Bounce is Your Guardrail. 88

    Achieving your target weight is a huge accomplishment! 88

Highway 44: What is Homeostasis? 90

    Tips to Achieve Homeostasis 90

Highway 45: Weight Fluctuation 92

Highway 46: Equilibrium, PAM, and PAW. 92

Highway 47: Blood Pressure—Simplified 94

Highway 48: Use Your Imagination! 94

Highway 49: An Explanation of PAM and PAW 98

Highway 50: Your Clothing 100

Highway 51: Update Your Success Plan 100

    Write down what the new you wants in your life: 100

    Initial Plateau Time 102

Highway 52: Physique and Lifestyle 104

    Have you met your goals and do you have future goals? 104

Highway 53: Maintaining an Optimal Physique and Lifestyle 106

Highway 54: Take Control of Your Health 108

Highway 55: Progress, Assessment, and Reassessment 110

    Below are a few issues and questions to consider: 110

    Get Organized and Stay Organized—Life & Lifestyle 110

Highway 56: Do Not Go to the Gym to Lose Weight! 112

    What is your revised weight loss plan? How often does it include exercise ?. 112

Highway 57: S.T.O.P. Is your Personal Action Plan 114

Highway 58: Tips for Success 116

    Challenges 118

    Victory Lane 118

Highway 59: Choose to Go to the Moon 120

Highway 60: Your STEM Highway to Wellness 122

Highway 61: The Winner's Circle—Forensic Wellness® Conclusion 124

Highways 62 and 63: Share your STEM Wellness Highway Journey and Visit your destination 126

Highway 64: A New Vision 128

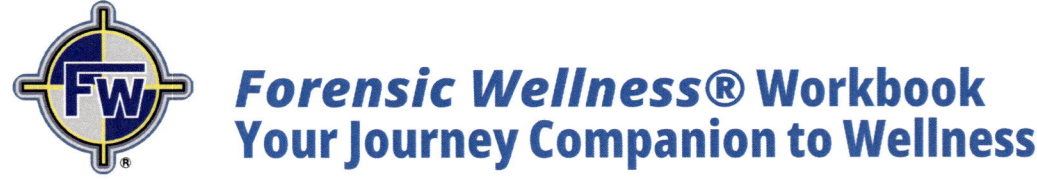

Welcome!
Highway 1: Why Highways Instead of Chapters?

Highways are more complex than chapters. Weight gain, weight loss, and a lifelong plan for weight control are comparable to interstate highway systems and signage around the country because of the complexity and challenges to safely reaching your destination.

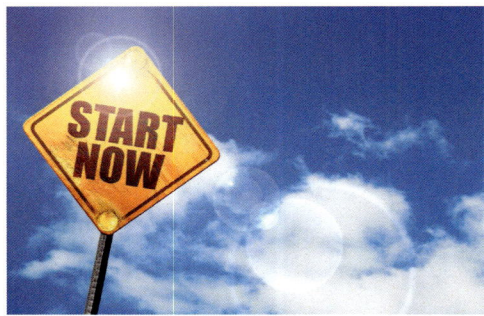

Go Forward Proactively—Your Highway To Wellness

Weight control, weight loss, and wellness are like a series of highways.

List the thoughts and challenges you may have about this journey below. It is important for you to be honest for this to work!

_____
_____
_____
_____
_____
_____
_____
_____
_____
_____

Forensic Wellness® Workbook
Your Journey Companion to Wellness

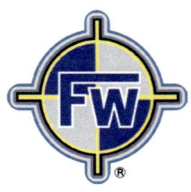

Forensic Wellness® Workbook
Your Journey Companion to Wellness

Your Story
Highway 2: Forensic STEM Wellness & Weight Loss = Train Your Mind to Lose Weight Permanently

Making the decision to focus on your long-term outcome of losing weight is important. To be successful, you must change your day-to-day behavior. This is an implementable wellness plan for your mind. Enjoy the journey to wellness. You have a lifetime ahead of you.

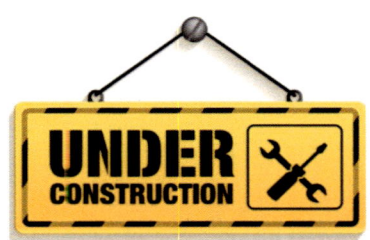

How Do I Do This?

Losing weight today is difficult. You know that a healthy lifestyle and eating healthy are important to achieve successful weight loss. If you have tried repeatedly to lose weight, but have not been successful, your plan did not work. Excess weight is the physical outcome of your thoughts and actions, or it could be ignoring what you have been taught or already know.

Change Your Story—Change Your Lifestyle

A successful journey includes four key terms: 1) Forensic, 2) STEM, 3) Wellness, and 4) Weight Loss. These terms come together in a simple scientific way. This is an implementable plan that successfully deals with today's complex and evolving world of life and personal health.

1. Forensic: a legally defensible position based on logic and available information
2. STEM: broad term to bring together these academic disciplines
3. Wellness: your objective
4. Weight Loss: the product of Wellness

How Do I See Myself?

Often, you may go on fad diets, lose a few pounds, then gain them right back. The **Forensic Wellness®** plan goes deeper than other diets including lifestyle, thought patterns and eating habits. This is a journey to examine your lifestyle, thought patterns, and eating habits—a strategy to learn about why you eat what you do. This is your workbook to write down your story.

Forensic Wellness® Workbook
Your Journey Companion to Wellness

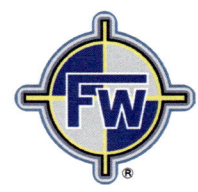

***Forensic Wellness®* Workbook**
Your Journey Companion to Wellness

ACT!

A: ACTION—What actions will you take today to lose weight and get healthy? Make a list of the first 4 actions you're going to take to get healthy and lose weight. Then do them!

_____

_____

_____

_____

C: CONNECT—Connect with your innermost feelings about food. Each time you eat, write down what you ate and why you ate it.

_____

_____

_____

_____

T: TIME—Today is the first day of your journey to a new healthy future. Mark this date down in your journal. This is the day you begin moving in a new and more healthy direction. This is the day you took control of not just your weight, but the direction of your life.

_____

_____

_____

_____

Forensic Wellness® Workbook
Your Journey Companion to Wellness

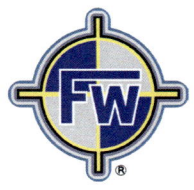

Highway 3: Let's Get Started! What is Wellness Visioning?

Believe: You Have What It Takes to Do This

Key Terms

- **STEM**—Science, Technology, Engineering, and Math
- **Wellness**—The state of being in good health

Three Foundational Steps:

Step 1)   The MIND Diet

Step 2)   Weight Tracking and Food Measurement Scales

Step 3)   Go Forward Proactively–Implement Step 1 and Step 2

Forensic Wellness is a Lifestyle for the Mind, Body, and Soul!

What is the MIND Diet?

(Refer to Forensic Wellness® book)

Diet for The Mind by Dr. Martha Clare Morris was published in 2017. Information about the MIND Diet will help you to better understand why it works so well.

Vision and Implementation

Let's vision and move to implementation. What is your current weight and what is your target weight?

Current Weight: _____   **Target Weight:** _____

An individual wants to achieve optimal health and wellness. This will include realistic weight loss and nutrition. To do this they will need to have an implementable weight loss and nutrition plan or diet.

This plan works because during the journey you change your lifestyle. You change how you think and feel about food and eating. Your goal is wellness.

What are your choices to fuel your body and improve brain function on your journey to wellness?

_____

_____

Forensic Wellness® Workbook
Your Journey Companion to Wellness

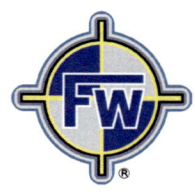

Forensic Wellness® Workbook
Your Journey Companion to Wellness

Lifestyle Tracker	Food	Exercise	Sleep	Successes Challenges
Monday				
Tuesday				
Wednesday				
Thursday				
Friday				
Saturday				
Sunday				

(This table can be copied & printed as needed.)

Forensic Wellness® Workbook
Your Journey Companion to Wellness

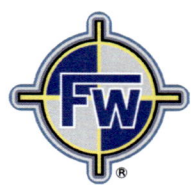

Highway 4: Your Challenges Today

Facts About Obesity

- The average American woman today weighs as much as the average 1960s male did.
- The average American adult has a weight gain of about 2/3 pound per year.
- At the moment, 40% of the American population age 20 and older is considered obese. About 70% are considered overweight.

Do you fall into this category?

Medical science has told us for decades that overweight and obese physiology leads to many health problems. Obesity dramatically increases the risk of developing serious medical conditions or diseases such as:

- Cancer
- Diabetes
- Coronary heart disease
- Osteoarthritis
- Sleep apnea
- High blood pressure
- Stroke
- Depression

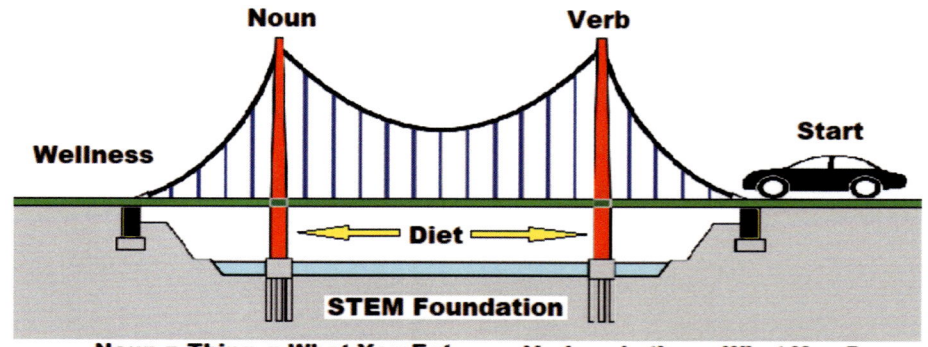

The U.S. Food and Drug Administration has implemented an added sugars disclosure on the "Nutrition Facts" label. This is part of a revamp of America's nutrition labeling rules as the nation battles obesity. There are also engineered food products that can addict your body to things like sugar. We will talk about all these things and how they affect your health.

My Current Personal Wellness Challenges

_____

_____

_____

Forensic Wellness® Workbook
Your Journey Companion to Wellness

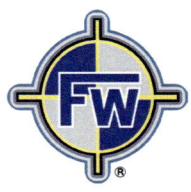

Forensic Wellness® Workbook
Your Journey Companion to Wellness

Highway 5: Weight Tracking and Food Measurement Scales

Eating three meals per day can reduce hunger and keep you full. If you eat three meals a day, then for two meals on one day, you need to figure out how many calories are in those two meals. That will tell you how many calories remain for your third meal.

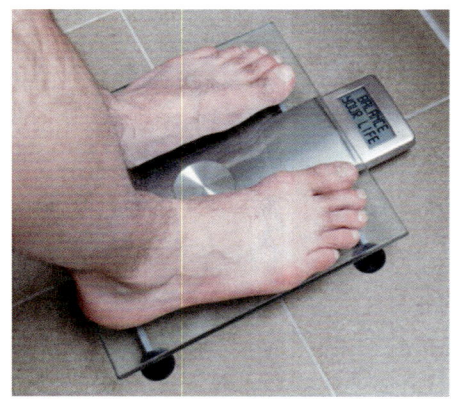

Today, we will begin in a new direction. We will take control of our health and our weight. You have a plan. You have the roadways to wellness. Let's retrain our thinking. The goal of achieving optimal health and weight is now within our reach.

It can be easier just to turn on the TV, grab a snack, and spend the evening watching a movie. Although it's fun and relaxing at first, over a period of time, it will lead to weight gain. Your muscles will get flabby. You'll get to the place where going to the mailbox each day makes you winded. Nobody likes the feeling of lethargy. We all hate looking at the scale to discover that we have gained weight.

My Progress: My Choices

_____
_____
_____
_____
_____
_____
_____
_____
_____
_____

Forensic Wellness® Workbook
Your Journey Companion to Wellness

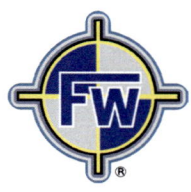

Highway 6: Challenges and A Plan

To be successful with weight control and weight loss today, it's vital to understand yourself. Overweight and obesity is a global and national problem. Your body is the most complex bio-mechanical machine on the planet. Food and drink are biologically and chemically turned into internal energy sources. Internal energy powers thought, mobility, and physical well-being.

The **Forensic Wellness®** plan is prepared and presented as a personally implementable plan. Here are the three specific areas of the **Forensic Wellness®** plan for both males and females, to stay fit for life:

1. Global/national overweight and obesity problem
2. Your body as a unique and complex biological machine
3. Your personal weight loss and weight control plan and lifestyle change.

Document and track challenges and successes as you implement these target areas.

_____

_____

_____

_____

_____

_____

_____

Spectator or Participant?

Becoming a participant means that you get involved at the most basic level. You have something valuable to gain by succeeding in this challenge. You can learn to train your mind and body to look at food in a different way.

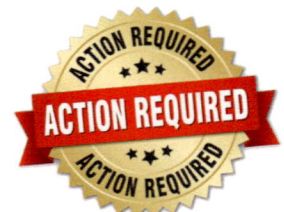

Forensic Wellness® Workbook
Your Journey Companion to Wellness

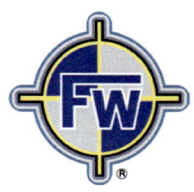

We want to have a healthy relationship with food. So let's talk about some of the ways that people develop UNHEALTHY relationships with food:

- Substituting it for love
- Emotional eating—using it to make ourselves feel better
- Eating when we're bored and just don't have anything better to do
- Stress
- For comfort
- Binge eating

A regular eating plan is the best solution to overeating.

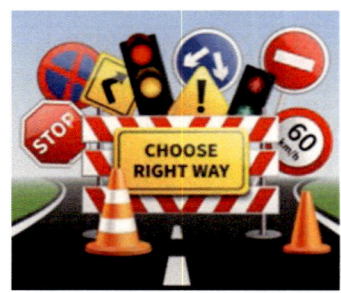

- Breakfast
- (Optional mid-morning snack)
- Lunch
- Afternoon snack
- Evening meal
- Evening Snack

The *Forensic Wellness®* plan will identify unhealthy food relationships that we may have. It will help us to retrain our thinking in this area. It will show us how to take control of our body. With your mind in control, your feelings and emotions will not control the way we live or eat.

What is your meal plan schedule? Are you losing or gaining weight?

_____
_____
_____
_____
_____

Forensic Wellness® Workbook
Your Journey Companion to Wellness

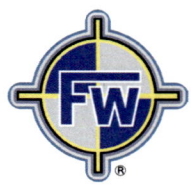

Highway 7: What Does STEM Mean?

STEM stands for:

S—Science: There's real science behind how our bodies use calories for nutrition and fuel.

T—Technology: We have the technology today to identify what causes obesity.

E—Engineering: The human body has evolved over thousands and millions of years. How you gather food and what you eat has evolved.

M—Math: If you eat more calories each day than your body requires for fuel, then you'll gain weight.

How many calories do you consume each day? _____

What is your implementable plan?

_____
_____
_____
_____

What are your thoughts and feelings as you institute your plan?

_____
_____
_____
_____
_____

Forensic Wellness® Workbook
Your Journey Companion to Wellness

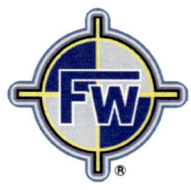

Highway 8: Realistic Weight Control

Let's work through the rules of calorie and nutrition to put in place your plan to achieve your target weight. The STEM plan is not quick weight loss. The STEM plan is a lifelong weight achievement plan. You can achieve your target weight. You can make corrections before gaining excess weight.

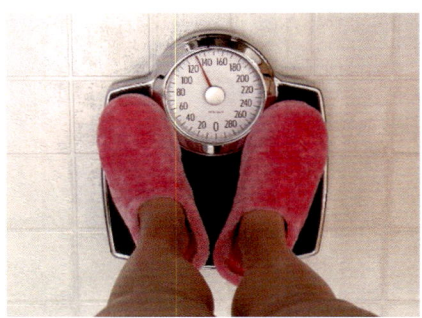

STEM To Lose Weight

To lose weight, your daily calorie intake must be less than the number of calories your body requires. (Review Highway 8 in the *Forensic Wellness®* book for an example of my typical breakfast and approximate calorie count.)

The U.S. Food and Drug Administration (FDA) uses 2,000-calorie diet as a typical daily example. Your individual number would likely be greater or less.

- Total daily calories in three meals - 940
- FDA typical daily calories - 2000
- Calorie difference - 1060
- Simplified calorie difference - 1000

Mathematically Calculating Weight Loss

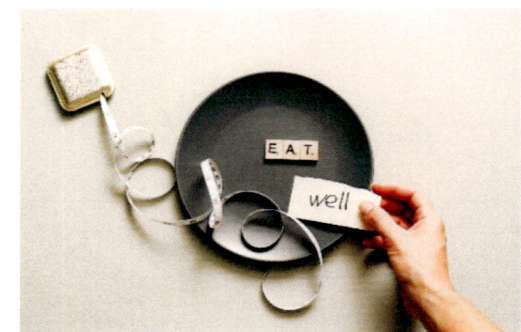

- Simplified calorie difference - 1000
- Calories in a pound of fat - 3500
- Daily weight loss: approximate 1/3 pound
- In 3 days, you would lose 1 pound
- In 30 days, you would lose 10 pounds

How do these FDA guidelines mirror your calorie intake?

_____

_____

_____

Forensic Wellness® Workbook
Your Journey Companion to Wellness

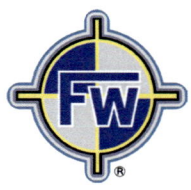

Your Plan for Weight Control

How the STEM Plan Can Help

Achieving weight loss is not simple. If it were easy, then there would not be a global obesity problem. Congratulations on your decision to take charge of your health now!

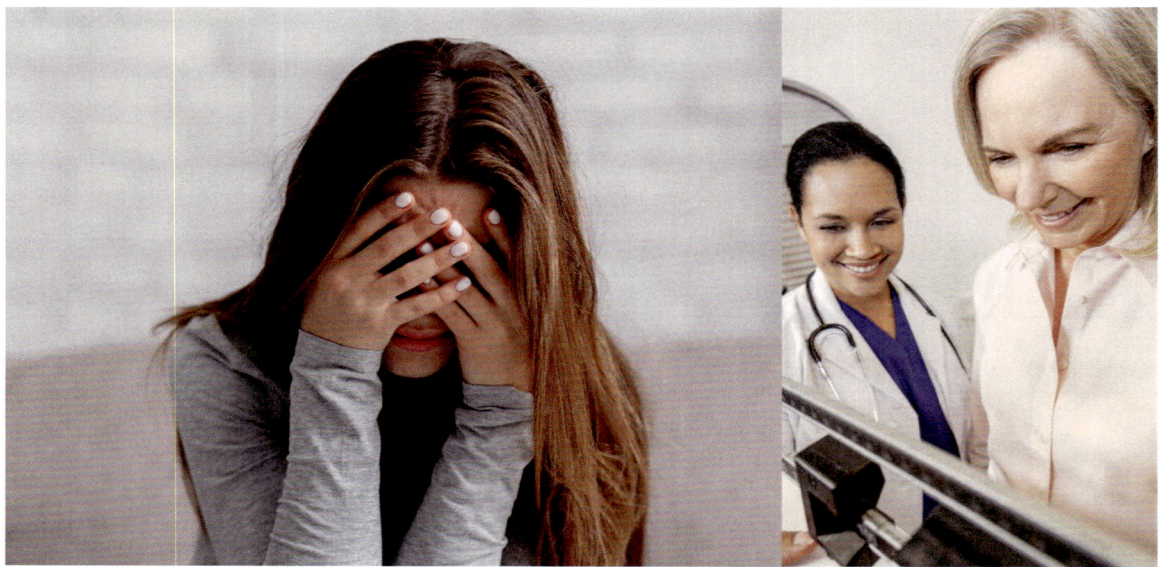

The STEM plan brings together three things:

1. Your vision of yourself
2. A realistic daily calorie number associated with nutritious foods that you eat
3. A personal STEM method to stick with your daily calorie number

In the STEM plan, you establish a personal target daily calorie number. If 2,000 is your calorie number and you consume 2,100, you are going to gain weight. If your calorie number is 1,900, you will lose weight.

How has the STEM Plan simplified your diet plan?

_____

_____

_____

Forensic Wellness® Workbook
Your Journey Companion to Wellness

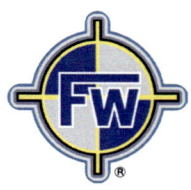

Highway 9: Critical Chain to Success

There's a formula in life for everything we do. For every journey, there is a starting point. There are stops along the way. Finally, there is a destination.

Below are our 10 steps toward improved health and wellness.

1. Proactive decision to lose weight
2. Establish target weight
3. One-day eating and calorie documentation
4. Establish initial timeline objective
5. Embark on the Weight Loss Highway
6. Weight loss rate (pounds/time)
7. Weight loss timeline—update/reassess
8. Transition to weight equilibrium
9. Weight Bounce
10. Arrive at a new mental attitude, physique, lifestyle, and wellness

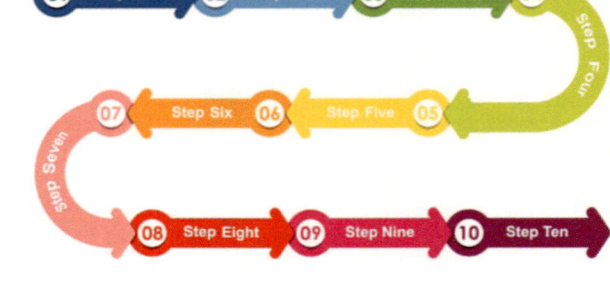

How to Arrive at the Number of Calories Your Body Requires Each Day

The number of calories you need to maintain health differs with age and activity level. Adult males generally need 2,000-3,000 calories per day to maintain weight. Adult females need around 1,600–2,400 calories according to the U.S. Department of Health.

What is your age? _____ **What are your daily calories to maintain?** _____

Are You on Track?

_____

_____

_____

_____

Forensic Wellness® Workbook
Your Journey Companion to Wellness

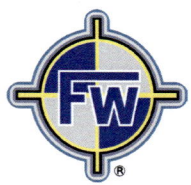

Forensic Wellness® Workbook
Your Journey Companion to Wellness

Highway 10: Your Specific Goals

To achieve any goal, you must know where you're headed and what it will take to get there. Essential elements to reach your goal include:

- Weight loss goal
- Game plan to get there
- Specific actions to take
- Checks and balances system

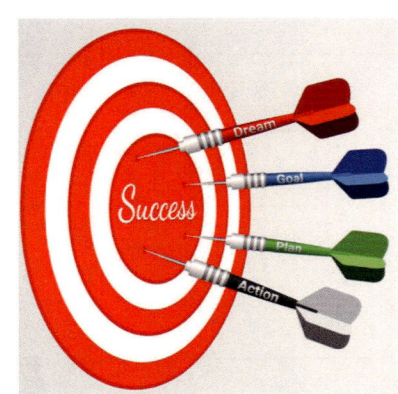

Your challenge is to achieve your goal. You should be doing this for yourself first, then for your loved ones.

Identify Your Target Weight and a Timeline: Be Realistic and Conservative.

_____

_____

_____

_____

_____

Cognitive Behavioral Therapy (CBT)

Each time you think about the bad habit or food, stop yourself. Close your eyes and focus on something else. Focus on a beautiful pond with blue water and green trees. Think calming thoughts. Recall favorite memories. Take a few deep breaths. Imagine a world where you are in control of your destiny.

- Step One: Imagine the outcome you desire.
- Step Two: Write down the steps to get there.
- Step Three: Take the first step.
- Step Four: Initiate a checks and balances system that informs you if you stray off-course.

Retrain your brain to believe that it IS possible because you are going to do it.

Forensic Wellness® Workbook
Your Journey Companion to Wellness

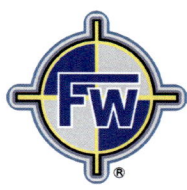

Highway 11: Selected Diets Backed by Science

Some diets have been scientifically studied and are effective in promoting health. These diets include the Mediterranean, DASH and MIND diets.

- The **Mediterranean diet** is a foundation for healthy diets.
- The **DASH** diet stands for Dietary Approaches to Stop Hypertension.
- The **MIND** diet stands for Mediterranean-DASH Intervention for Neurodegenerative Delay.

The MIND diet includes parts of the Mediterranean and DASH diets. A specific goal was to reduce dementia and the decline of brain health that can occur with age.

Guidelines for the MIND diet
(may be found in the *Forensic Wellness®* book)

The MIND diet and healthy habits like exercise, not smoking and, adequate sleep may have an effect on cognition. Benefits include heart health and reduced risk of cardiovascular disease and diabetes. Both heart and cardiovascular disease are risk factors for Alzheimer's disease. Many other factors impact the development of Alzheimer's disease; at this time there is no known cure.

What foods from the MIND Diet are you including in your diet plan?

_____

_____

_____

_____

_____

_____

_____

Forensic Wellness® Workbook
Your Journey Companion to Wellness

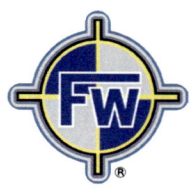

Highway 12: Think Globally but Act Locally and Personally

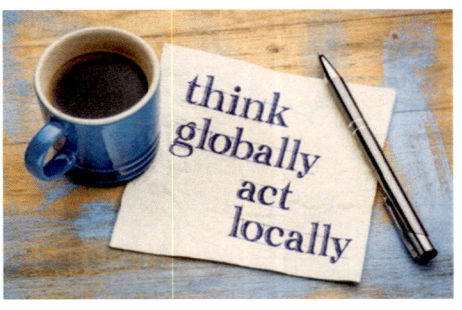

Your choices when shopping are critical. What you bring home is what you and your family will eat. Healthy eating begins with logical healthy food selections. That means bringing home fresh fruits and vegetables for your family to consume.

Obesity was uncommon 100 years ago. One of the reasons was that most Americans lived in rural communities where they grew much of the food they ate. They raised their own beef, pork, and chicken. There was no such thing as running to the grocery store to pick up ice cream, snack cakes and carbonated beverages. There were no fast food places to get a bag of hamburgers.

Do you notice a difference in your thinking as you are shopping? Do you make different choices in restaurants yet? Have you experienced any differences in how you feel about yourself, your weight, and the image you see in the mirror?

_____
_____
_____
_____
_____
_____
_____
_____
_____

Forensic Wellness® Workbook
Your Journey Companion to Wellness

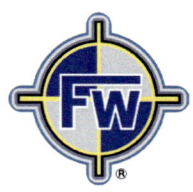

Highway 13: Your Personal Weigh-In

Tracking your weight loss over time starts with a weigh-in. Knowing your current weight and checking your weight daily is critical. These are essential elements of your weight loss plan.

Your Scale and Tracking System

A good tracking system is essential. You wouldn't go off on a trip in your car without knowing where you're headed. To get to a destination, you need a clear idea of the starting point and the ending point. You need a direct route to make the best use of your time and other resources.

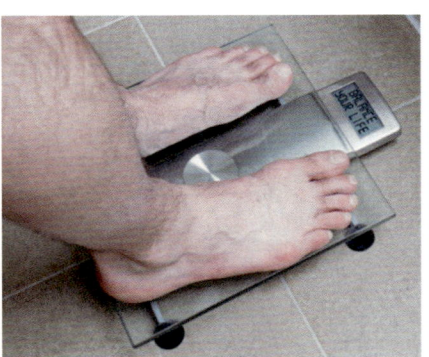

Your Weight Loss Tracking: A Starting Point

Month/Year:

Sunday	Monday	Tuesday	Wednesday	Thursday	Friday	Saturday

(This table can be copied & printed as needed.)

Forensic Wellness® Workbook
Your Journey Companion to Wellness

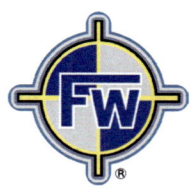

***Forensic Wellness*® Workbook**
Your Journey Companion to Wellness

Your Story: 1) Have you ever been at your perfect weight and body shape in your lifetime? 2) What was going on in your life at that time that was good? 3) When is the first time you recall being dissatisfied with your weight, appearance, or you felt you outgrew your clothes? What was happening in your life at that time? 4) Did you ever get back to your desired weight? How long did it take? What did you do differently? 5) What do you think will change in your life when you acheive your desired weight?

_____

_____

_____

_____

_____

_____

_____

_____

_____

_____

_____

_____

_____

_____

_____

Forensic Wellness® Workbook
Your Journey Companion to Wellness

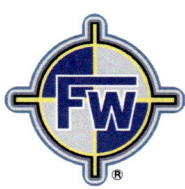

Highway 14: Key Steps to Successful Weight Loss

Let's begin by asking ourselves 4 important questions:

1. Why am I overweight?
2. How can I lose weight in a healthy manner?
3. How can I maintain my target weight and will my family and friends help or hamper my journey?
4. Will my new weight loss plan be sustainable for my physique for the long term?

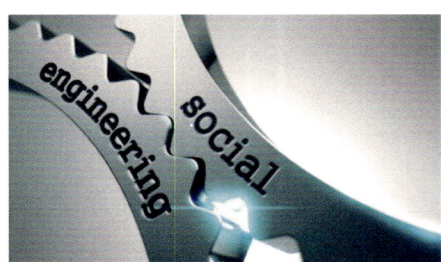

Down deep, we all want to be happy, healthy and look our best. We all know that being overweight can cause a multitude of health issues. **Tell yourself every day that you're about to get happy and healthy.** You're about to lose those excess pounds and life will be fun and amazing once you do, because you'll be able to do all the things that you've dreamed of doing. Your clothes will fit better. Your confidence level will rise. You'll take the world by storm!

What challenge(s) are blocking you from being HAPPY?

_____
_____
_____
_____
_____
_____
_____
_____
_____

Forensic Wellness® Workbook
Your Journey Companion to Wellness

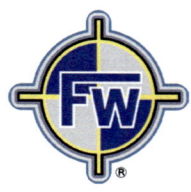

Highway 15: Question #1—Why Are You Overweight?

Now, write down some truthful answers. Be honest with yourself. Do not be embarrassed or ashamed to admit certain things about yourself. You do not need to share this with anyone. This is the time to get REAL with yourself. When the answers are recorded here and you're satisfied that these are true reasons, then say or think about each one: "I am overweight because...."

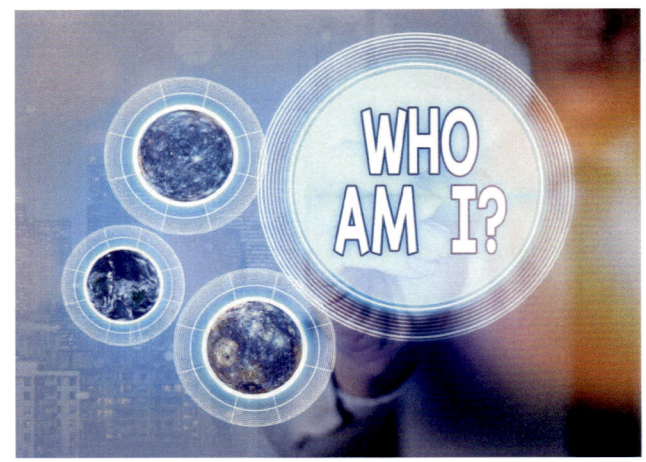

Sometimes the most important step in dealing with a problem in our own lives is to admit that it exists. If necessary, give it a name, a shape, a form ... describe the problem in your own words.

Your Real Answers:

_____
_____
_____
_____
_____
_____
_____
_____
_____
_____
_____

Forensic Wellness® Workbook
Your Journey Companion to Wellness

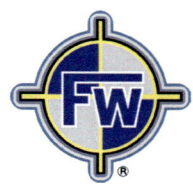

Highway 16: Question #2—Can I Lose Weight in a Healthy Manner?

Think about all the fad diets you have heard about. Many dieters have been on a roller coaster ride up and down, or slammed back and forth.

Some of these diets will result in weight loss. Many people get off the diet, and gradually gain the weight back. Why? Because the person never changed their mindset about eating. For permanent weight control you have to change your eating habits. If a person goes back to the old style of eating, the weight will come back. Each time the weight comes back, it becomes harder to lose weight the next time.

Some Reasons Why You Might Overeat?

Here is a list to refresh your memory. Feel free to add to this list:
- Substituting it for love
- Emotional eating, using it to make ourselves feel better
- Eating when we're bored and just don't have anything better to do
- Stress
- For comfort
- Binge eating

My thoughts on how I can maintain my target weight:

_____
_____
_____
_____
_____
_____
_____

Forensic Wellness® Workbook
Your Journey Companion to Wellness

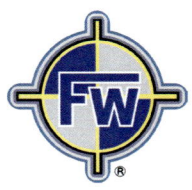

Forensic Wellness® Workbook
Your Journey Companion to Wellness

Highway 17: Maintaining target weight: How family and friends may affect your journey

Most of us do want to be happy, healthy and prosperous. Most of us care what we look like in our clothes. We desire to live our best life. If extra weight is holding you back, it is time for action. If extra weight is preventing you from accomplishing some dreams, it is time for action.

Talk openly and candidly with friends and family members about these issues. It can truly make a difference in how well you do on the program. Give yourself every possible chance for success because you are worth it! You're worth the extra time, effort, and hard work. *(Some example questions you may ask them are: Have you noticed when I first began to gain weight? Was I happy or unhappy with my life, job, or relationships? Do you remember if I used food to bring me comfort?)*

Results of your feedback:

_____

_____

_____

_____

_____

_____

_____

_____

_____

_____

Forensic Wellness® Workbook
Your Journey Companion to Wellness

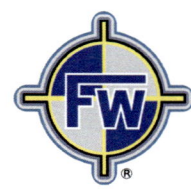

Highway 18: Sustaining Your Physique

What is your current personal image? Developing a target vision provides reinforcement every time you look into the mirror. Personal image is central to making the hard-minded decisions that must be made on a daily basis to reach or maintain your personal image.

What type of physique is your goal? This may be an easier mindset to understand than reaching a specific weight. Look in the mirror and assess your physique.

- What do you look like today?
- What would you change?
- What would you like your body to look like for the rest of your life?

Write down your answers below.

_____
_____
_____
_____
_____
_____
_____
_____
_____
_____

Forensic Wellness® Workbook
Your Journey Companion to Wellness

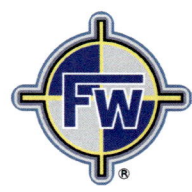

Highway 19: STEM Plan Reality vs. Self-Delusion

The "Secret" of the STEM plan is that it provides logical building blocks of an implementable plan. This plan will assist you in making daily decisions, which will result in weight loss.

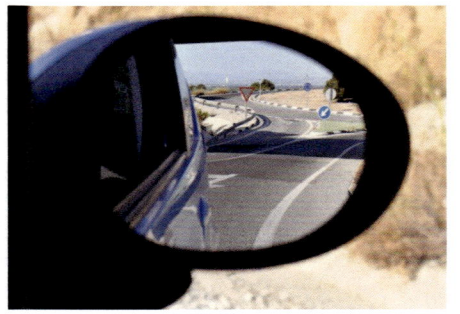

Quick and massive weight loss is not part of the STEM plan. If you are looking for quick/big numbers, there are plenty of diets that provide this. Quick fad weight loss programs may not be healthy or successful. If they were successful then a lot more people would be skinny. Right? There would not be an obesity crisis all over the globe.

Record your thoughts below.

_____
_____
_____
_____
_____
_____
_____
_____
_____
_____
_____

Forensic Wellness® Workbook
Your Journey Companion to Wellness

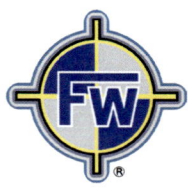

Forensic Wellness® Workbook
Your Journey Companion to Wellness

Highway 20: A Sustainable Weight Loss Plan

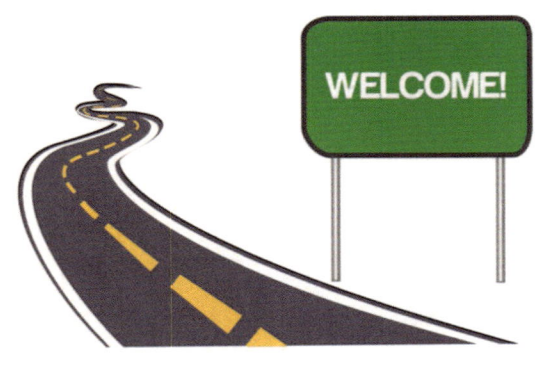

Your challenge is to retrain your brain! What we are doing here is retraining the way we think and respond to certain issues. In the past, you may have turned to food as a substitute for love or a stressful life situation. We're not going to do that anymore.

Encourage yourself! You can do this! Think this and say it out loud: "I can do this! I'm losing weight and taking control of my health."

Remember ... this is a journey to retrain the way to think, feel, and respond to food. As your relationship with food changes, your relationships with people will change, too. Expect this to happen and be prepared.

Successes and challenges you've had so far:

_____
_____
_____
_____
_____
_____
_____
_____
_____

Forensic Wellness® Workbook
Your Journey Companion to Wellness

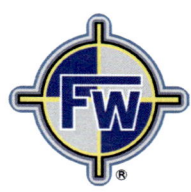

Highway 21: The Real You

Your height to weight relationship is important. If twice your waist measurement is equal to or more than your height, in inches, you are overweight.

Take your waist measurement at belly button and suck in stomach to get a good number. Now double that number in inches. Is it more than the number of inches you are tall?

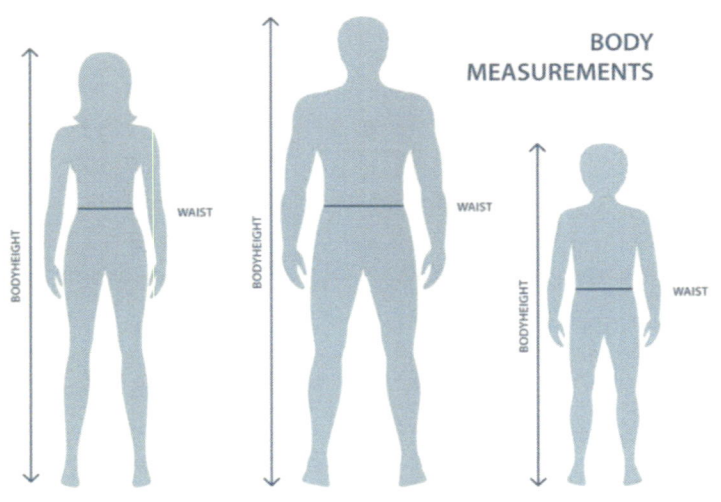

Example 1:

Waist–32 inches [32" x 2 = 64"]

Height–60 inches [5'0" x 12 = 60"]

64 inches is more than 60 inches.

Calculation: You are overweight.

Example 2:

Waist–32 inches [32" x 2 = 64"]

Height–72 inches [6'0" x 12 = 72"]

64 inches is less than 72 inches.

Calculation: You are not overweight.

The entire process starts in your brain with your thought process. It's all about how you think about food, yourself, and your world. What you eat is the initial critical link in weight loss.

How do you fit into the height to weight ratio?

_____
_____
_____
_____
_____
_____

Forensic Wellness® Workbook
Your Journey Companion to Wellness

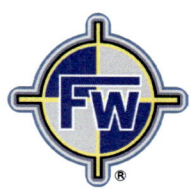

Highway 22: Healthy Food Costs

If you train your mind and body, good things can happen. Foods such as tomatoes, spinach, grapes, blueberries, strawberries, broccoli, and nuts are good for you. With good foods you can lose weight. Benefits associated with getting healthy do not necessarily cost a fortune. Include healthy fats in your eating plan. Healthy fats include avocados, olive oil, coconut oil, walnuts, and chia seeds. Just about all nuts and seeds are good for you. Dark chocolate is a healthy fat that can also satisfy your need for something decadent and sweet. Salmon and Mahi Mahi are healthy foods with Omega-3 fatty acids.

Ideas for Healthy, Low-Cost Meals (may be found in the *Forensic Wellness*® book)

How do these examples fit into your meal plan? List the foods you currently have in your meal plan:

Breakfast:

_____

_____

_____

Lunch:

_____

_____

_____

Dinner:

_____

_____

_____

Forensic Wellness® Workbook
Your Journey Companion to Wellness

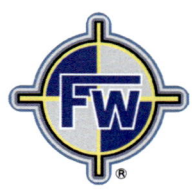

Forensic Wellness® Workbook
Your Journey Companion to Wellness

Highway 23: Take Suggestions and Make Decisions

You are in control of your weight loss, one day and one bite at a time. Your brain is your personal Chief Executive Officer. You can make the right choices—the good—decisions you need to make each day. Here are some of your daily CEO responsibilities.

- Activity Center
- Propulsion
- Bio Factory
- Weight Control
- Mental Control
- Personal Control
- Calorie Control
- Weight Control
- Activity Control
- Brain Control

This program encourages you to take control of your life, to make better decisions, and to resist those urges to snack on unhealthy foods. Get on a more regimented schedule especially when it comes to meals. Don't wait until you're starving to eat. There's a good chance you'll eat the wrong things and regret it later. Make sure to always have healthy snack foods around such as nuts, grapes, berries, and fresh fruit. Be sure to make healthy daily choices in these five areas.

➢ Daily and weekly scheduled activity _____

➢ Restaurants, and foods _____

➢ Supermarket, and fast foods _____

➢ Home food, cooking, and snacks _____

➢ Soda and energy drinks _____

Forensic Wellness® Workbook
Your Journey Companion to Wellness

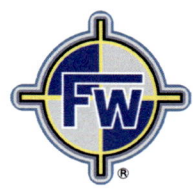

Highway 24: Is Achieving Your Weight Loss the Equivalent of the Moon Shot?

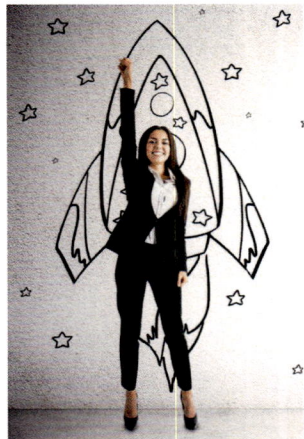

How difficult is it to lose weight? Remember that it has taken years to get your body to its current shape. Achieving your weight and physique goals, logically, will take time.

To reach your weight loss destination you need to travel many highways. Reaching your destination of weight and physique is not an easy task or challenge. But you're worth the hard work. Your life and future will be amazing now that you've got control.

Your Precision Preparation
You need a Personal Clear Sight Plan for Weight Loss:

_____

_____

_____

_____

Vision Implementation
- ➢ Your Personal Weight Loss Plan requires Vision and Implementation in a Logical and Doable Manner
- ➢ Vision Implementation Added to What Seems Logical and Doable, Yields Your Weight Loss Plan

_____

_____

_____

_____

Forensic Wellness® Workbook
Your Journey Companion to Wellness

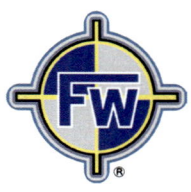

Highway 25: Dieting Is Not as Far as Away as the Moon

Each eating activity has two choices — high calorie or lower calorie, good nutrition or poor nutrition. Your conflict? Which calorie decision to make — high vs lower calorie? Nutritional vs Unhealthy.

Once you have lost some weight and started feeling better, don't forget to acknowledge and feel great about your weight loss success. It is not easy, but you did it!

How Difficult Is It to Lose Weight?

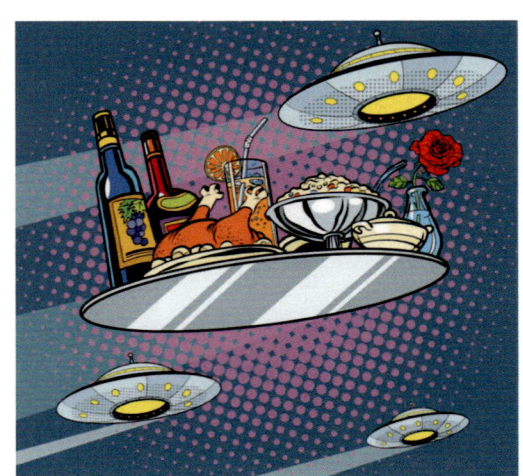

Many would say that they think it is about as difficult as sending a man or woman to the moon. NASA's Apollo moon program consumed up to 4.5% of the U.S. budget between 1960 and 1972. This is a valuation of $176 billion 2022 dollars. Achieving weight loss requires participation, planning, dedication, time, and modest resources (when compared to the moon initiative)

How difficult has it been to lose weight for you?

___
___
___
___
___
___
___
___
___

Forensic Wellness® Workbook
Your Journey Companion to Wellness

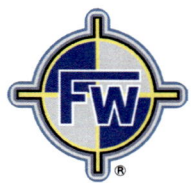

Highway 26: Lose and Maintain Your Desired Weight

This is a three-step process. It begins with transitioning your body through weight stabilization. This is the first critical step to weight control and weight loss. To say that this is a tough step would be accurate. If you are unable to stabilize your weight, you will not be able to lose weight and keep it off. Stabilization means that your daily calorie count is equal to the calorie count your body needs.

An equation could be written as:
Calories In = Calories Needed.

Stabilization of calorie count is the First Objective associated with achieving Your Goal.

Your Thoughts:

_____

_____

_____

_____

_____

_____

_____

_____

_____

Forensic Wellness® Workbook
Your Journey Companion to Wellness

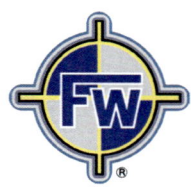

Highway 27: Set a Target!

With the target on the wall, you know the exact direction associated with Your Goal. Every movement you make toward Your Goal brings you closer to success.

The pathway is not straight. Every decision you make associated with Calories In = Calories Needed represents a number. Each decision moves you away or toward Your Goal.

What is your weight loss target goal?

_____

_____

_____

Highway 28: Determine the Right Calorie Number

You must develop a personal baseline associated with your daily calorie count. Everyone is different so you will need to come up with your own number. To provide a starting point associated with calories, let's use some basic numbers. Calorie counting requires keeping track of numbers.

Here are three generally accepted calorie numbers to use for reference. 2,000 calories per day for men 1,600 for women, and 3,500 calories associated with one pound of fat. Your actual daily number to maintain your body is the Basal Metabolic Rate (BMR).

You can enter your physical data to arrive at a calorie calculation for your body.

BMR (kcal)
1652

What is your BMR? _____

Your Current Calories Per Day? _____

Target Calories Per Day? _____

Calories to Cut to Stay at Target Calories Per Day? _____

Forensic Wellness® Workbook
Your Journey Companion to Wellness

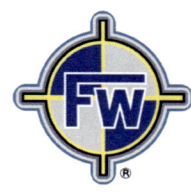

Highway 29: For Women Only

Every woman knows that it's more difficult for her to lose weight than for the average man. I believe this may have a lot to do with hormones. Women have many more hormones than men and these hormones tend to fluctuate almost on a daily basis. That's why weight loss is often more challenging for women than for men.

If you're a female and feel that your hormones may be fluctuating wildly, causing you to gain weight, then see your OB/GYN. He or she can run tests to see where you're at as far as hormones go. Your doctor will recommend a course of action to get the hormone situation under control.

Your experience(s):

_____

_____

_____

_____

_____

_____

_____

_____

_____

_____

_____

_____

Forensic Wellness® Workbook
Your Journey Companion to Wellness

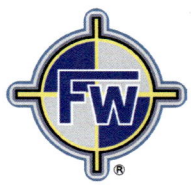

Highway 30: For Women & Men

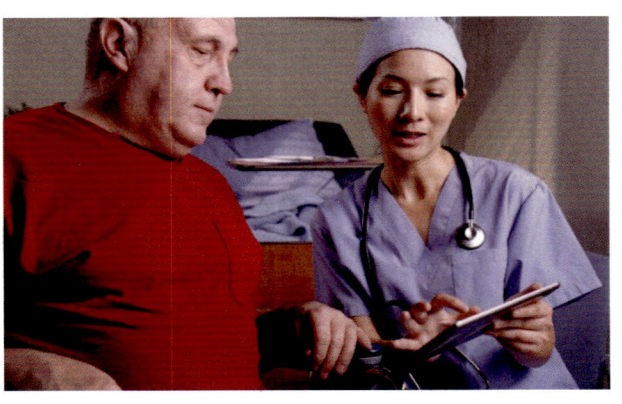

Sometimes there are other medical reasons why someone may not be able to lose weight. The most common is a thyroid condition.

Your metabolic rate and thyroid are related. Unexplained changes in body weight may be indicative of thyroid trouble. Weight gain, with no changes in what you eat or your activity level, may indicate a thyroid problem. Changes in appetite, exercise, or stress level may suggest low thyroid hormone production. Excess thyroid production may also provoke weight loss for no clear reason.

For this book, we will assume that each person is in fairly good health. We also assume that there are no underlying medical conditions that impact your weight gain or loss. If your health is compromised, proactively speak with your physician.

Have you ever been tested for or diagnosed as having any kind of thyroid condition in the past 5–10 years? If so, how has it affected your weight loss?

_____
_____
_____
_____
_____
_____
_____
_____

Forensic Wellness® Workbook
Your Journey Companion to Wellness

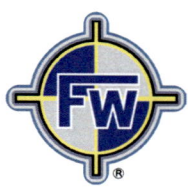

Highway 31: Commitment

Losing weight requires commitment, but so does getting an education or going to work each day. Once you make the decision to take control of your weight, think of it as a commitment to life-long wellness.

If you're married or have a partner, you've committed to make a life with another person. There are challenges to making a good relationship work. Maintaining a healthy body is no different. It will require work and dedication but you're worth it. You can extend your lifespan and improve your quality of life by staying healthy and in shape.

Make a commitment in the beginning of your journey and stay with it. Yes, there will be temptations to cheat. If you want this relationship with your body to remain healthy, you must make some changes.

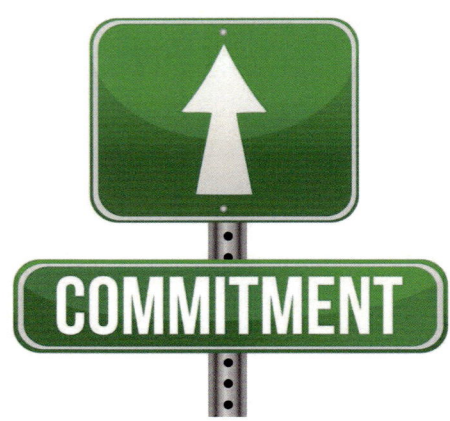

What is your Level of Commitment?

_____
_____
_____
_____
_____
_____
_____
_____
_____
_____

Forensic Wellness® Workbook
Your Journey Companion to Wellness

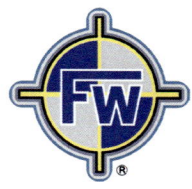

Highway 32: Equilibrium Value

Once you have your BMR, you will know your daily calorie number. Getting a viable number for Equilibrium Value (EV) can be achieved in one of two ways. Historically, for women and men the number is 1,600 and 2,000 calories, respectively. However, this metric does not necessarily take into account age, metabolism, or exercise, but it does represent a baseline number for ease of explanation.

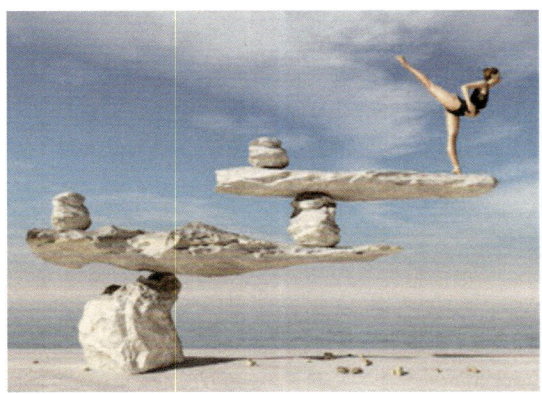

Using a calorie calculator, you can arrive at a more accurate number. As you progress down the wellness highway, you will become more familiar with your body. You will assess how it works, and how well it responds to exercise and changes in your eating patterns.

You will learn and analyze your own lifestyle. You will analyze strengths and weaknesses. You will gain a better global understanding for your own personal Equilibrium Value.

You will develop new and more healthy relationships with food.

How has this changed your perspective with what you consume?

_____
_____
_____
_____
_____
_____
_____
_____
_____

Forensic Wellness® Workbook
Your Journey Companion to Wellness

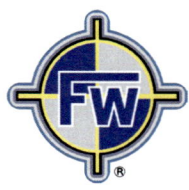

Highway 33: Critical Mass (CM) and Equilibrium Value (EV)

Very simply, CM is your ultimate weight target and it is sustained by your EV Equilibrium Value daily calorie intake. Therefore to maintain your ultimate desired weight, CM = EV.

To phrase it differently, if your desired weight target is 160 lb. and after getting to your target you have determined that 1,500 calories are required to maintain your weight, the equation would look like this:

$$CM = EV >>> 160 \text{ lb.} = 1{,}500 \text{ calories} >>> 160 = 1500$$

As long as your calorie intake remains at 1,500 then your weight will remain stable at 160 lb.

What is your target weight? _____

What is your calorie count to maintain your target weight? _____

Highway 34: WLC, WLM, and Bounce

Getting to target weight the first time is a huge wonderful moment. Reading your scale weight has validated all your dedication to achieving that magical number. Achieving that number means that you have entered a new phase of Weight Loss Control (WLC) and Weight Loss Monitoring (WLM).

WLC and WLM are the issues that most people grapple with. They can take off the weight but just not maintain it. Failure to remain at the target weight is the result of:

1. Not acknowledging the daily scale number
2. Reverting to higher calorie intake
3. After reaching Target Weight, your ups and downs are called "Bounce."

Your Thoughts:

_____

_____

_____

_____

Forensic Wellness® Workbook
Your Journey Companion to Wellness

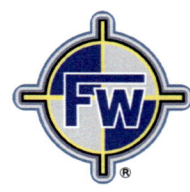

Highway 35: Stay on the Highway. Don't Exit to a Sideroad

You must remind yourself often that you're on a new pathway. You're not the same person anymore. You've chosen to live healthy and free of those extra pounds that thwart your happiness.

What is Your happiness level at Mile Marker Highway 35?

_____

_____

_____

_____

Highway 36: Meal Planning

Remember to plan for meals in advance. Every day, we have to eat. Even if you are simply having cereal for breakfast, be sure to have something on hand that's healthy. For lunch, try a tuna or turkey sandwich and bowl of vegetable soup. At dinner, make yourself a lean steak or hamburger patty, a sweet potato and a salad with minimal or no dressing.

It's important to eat at each meal, so it doesn't feel like you're starving yourself to death. At the same time, making healthier food choices will benefit you in so many ways. You will lose weight, but you'll also begin to have more energy. You'll feel better and you will feel more positive about your life. You are making proactive wellness decisions.

What Are Your Favorite Go-To Healthy Meals (Breakfast, Lunch, Dinner, and Snacks)?

_____

_____

_____

_____

Forensic Wellness® Workbook
Your Journey Companion to Wellness

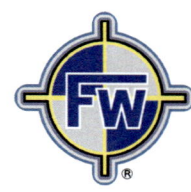

Highway 37: One-Day Calorie Count

These days, it's easy to get calorie and nutritional values from food containers and websites. It is important to keep a notebook handy for one day. **Keep track of your calories consumed each day**. This will make you more aware about what you eat and drink. Often, we eat a lot more than we realize. If you write it all down for one day, you will know exactly what you eat and the number of calories in each meal and for the day. You will have established a solid foundation about why you were overweight to start with.

What are your calorie counts for your 5 favorite foods?

_____
_____
_____
_____

Highway 38: Realistic Weight Loss Expectation & Plan

It may be possible to lose a pound a day or 30 pounds in a month. You'll have to change your eating habits and get more exercise.

Remember that it takes 3,500 calories to gain or lose a pound. **If you want to lose 30 pounds, then you'll have to eliminate 105,000 calories from your diet in one month's time.**

What is your weight loss expectation?

For such an aggressive weight loss plan, it is essential to consult your medical or nutritional advisor.

_____
_____
_____
_____

Forensic Wellness® Workbook
Your Journey Companion to Wellness

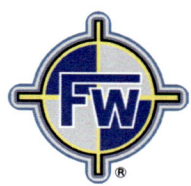

Highway 39: Personal Checklist

You Can Lose Weight

- You have proven that you can lose weight
- You can share your weight-loss success with others
- You can look at the results on the smartphone and computer
- You can discuss it with others
- You can take pride in your weight-loss success story

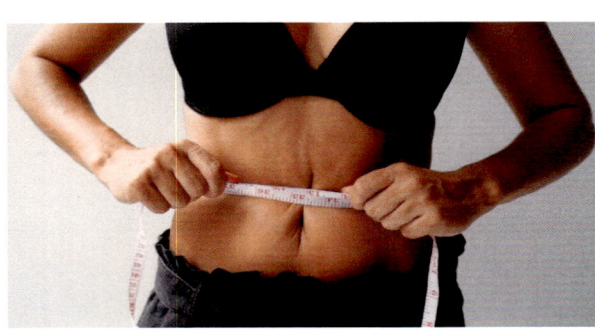

Personal and Honest Reality Check

You have to get personal about what you eat and how much you eat. Has your daily calorie burn changed any? Has it improved? The more active you are each day, the more calories you can consume. Of course, if you avoid consuming those calories, this will result in greater weight loss. Is your system regular or irregular? Consume enough fiber for good bowel health.

Go-To Foods

Have the right foods available and easy to consume. Don't make it difficult to eat healthy. Keep some carrots, celery, apples, grapes, strawberries, and such around for snacking. Dried fruits are delicious, nutritious and easy to eat; try cherries, mangoes, and apricots. Nuts are good for you too, especially pistachios, and mixed nuts.

Foods to Avoid Include:

- Sugar and sweeteners
- Soda
- Beer, wine, and mixed drinks
- Ice cream
- Candy bars
- Starches like pasta and potatoes
- All cheeses
- Hamburgers, hot dogs
- Anything fried
- Gravies
- High-calorie sauces
- High-calorie salad dressing

Forensic Wellness® Workbook
Your Journey Companion to Wellness

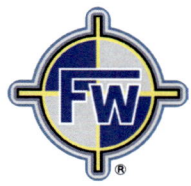

Which Items in the "Foods to Avoid" List Do You Eat Frequently?

_____
_____
_____
_____
_____
_____
_____
_____
_____
_____
_____
_____
_____
_____
_____
_____
_____

Highway 40: Math—Daily, Monthly, and Yearly Weight Loss

There are five key numbers for weight control and weight loss: 3500, 350, 0, 1, and 3. The largest number is 3,500. This is a critical number because there are 3,500 calories in a pound of fat. If you are going to reduce your fat weight by 1-pound, then you need to eliminate 3,500 calories.

This key relationship and calculation is a useful metric. Reduce your daily calorie intake by 10 calories to achieve a 1-pound weight loss in one year. (Calculation examples may be found in the *Forensic Wellness*® book.)

As you continue down this road of thought, you can logically see that if you reduce your calorie intake by just 100 calories per day, you can lose 10 times that much weight or 10 pounds in one year.

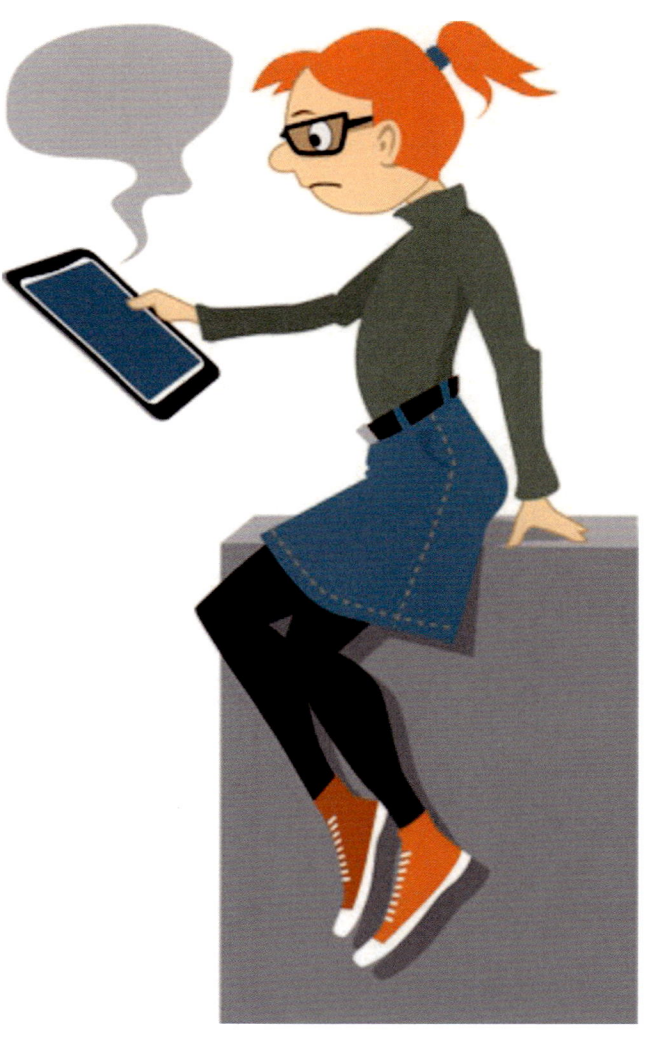

100 calories is equal to about:

1 slice of bread

2 slices of cheese

1 medium baked potato

2 small biscuits

A plain grilled hamburger with bun contains about 450 calories. A scoop of your favorite ice cream is typically about 150–300 calories. Large scoops of premium ice cream can reach 450 calories. There are 150 calories in one little hot dog. Add the bun and it's over 300 calories. There are around 200 calories in one cup of cooked rice. There are 200 calories in ½ cup of sausage gravy. A sausage and egg biscuit is 500 calories. A cup of mashed potatoes contains around 210 calories.

Forensic Wellness® Workbook
Your Journey Companion to Wellness

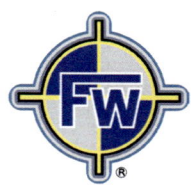

Forensic Wellness® Workbook
Your Journey Companion to Wellness

Highway 41: Math Utilization Areas

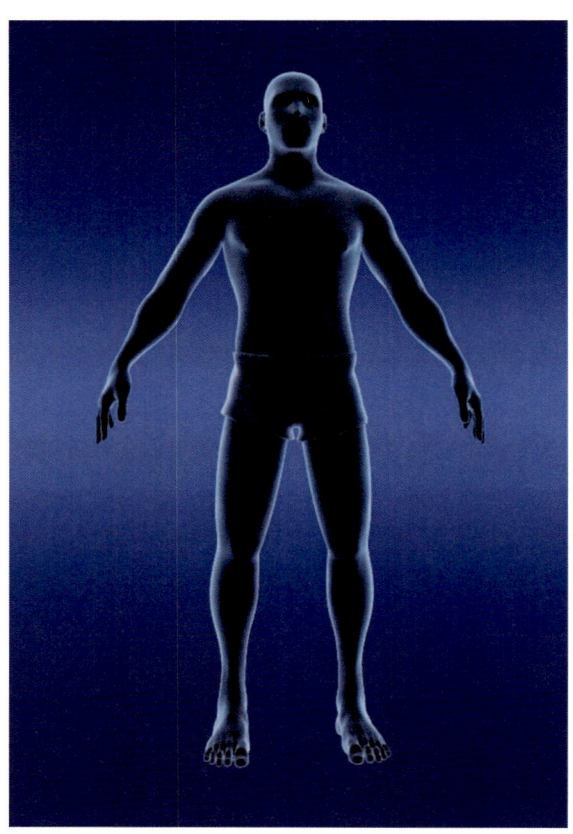

Weight Loss Tools
- Smart scale
- Computer
- Smartphone

Identify Potential "Slippery Slopes"
- Processed foods
- Advertising
- Restaurants
- Temptation

Proactive Decision Making
- Your body shape vision
- Start today, not tomorrow

Healthy Weight and Body
- Physical Skeleton Structure
- Weight Mass Structure
- Body Mass Index
- Portion Control
- Restaurant Menu Calorie Count
- Weight Fluctuation
- Personal Space

Your Daily, Monthly, and Yearly Weight Loss:

_____

_____

Forensic Wellness® Workbook
Your Journey Companion to Wellness

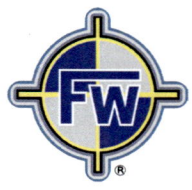

Highway 42: Social and Peer Pressure

To take weight off and keep it off requires stick-to-it-ive-ness. I might take that a step further and say that it requires hard-headedness.

To change one's lifestyle is never easy, especially if we're talking about eating habits. We learn our eating habits from the time we're born. Everything you know about eating is learned from your parents, siblings, friends, lifestyle—that's why it is so difficult to change.

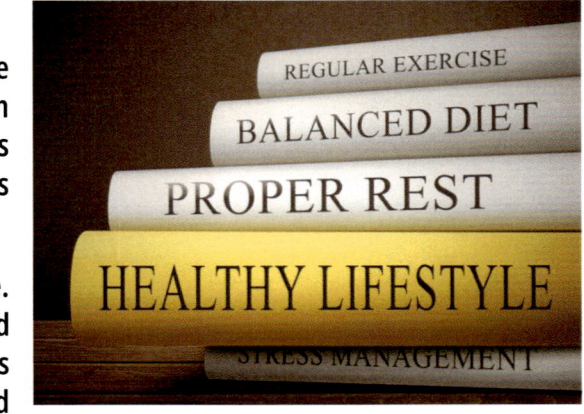

Changing what you eat represents a major lifestyle change. Changing what you eat and how much you eat affects you and everyone around you. Psychological and sociological pressures in life and society absolutely require that you have a solid understanding associated with the challenges of weight loss and maintaining that targeted weight.

How is social and peer pressure challenging your wellness journey? Are you being encouraged or discouraged by friends and family?

_____
_____
_____
_____
_____
_____
_____
_____
_____

Forensic Wellness® Workbook
Your Journey Companion to Wellness

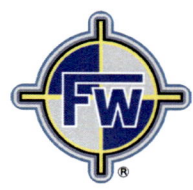

Highway 43: Target Weight Bounce is Your Guardrail

Achieving your target weight is a huge accomplishment!

Transitioning to a weight maintenance diet (WMD) will take time though. Whether you've lost 10 pounds or 50, moving around is easier. You feel better. Without those extra pounds, living your life doesn't require as much energy. But there are always temptations and sometimes we give in to them. Very quickly, you can gain several, 5, or 10 pounds again!

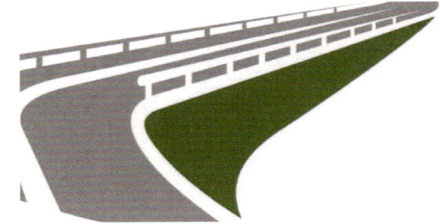

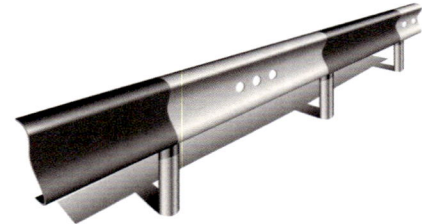

As you determine your target number of calories, there are a few variables to consider. The Target Number of calories is the number you do not want to go over. When you are losing weight or you have reached your target weight the term Bounce Range applies. This term uses your upper and lower numbers to establish guardrails. You have reached the Bounce phase of the *Forensic Wellness*® plan.

What is your target weight bounce?

_____
_____
_____
_____
_____
_____
_____
_____
_____

Forensic Wellness® Workbook
Your Journey Companion to Wellness

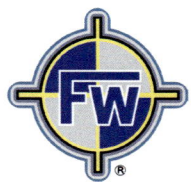

_____

_____

_____

_____

_____

_____

_____

_____

_____

_____

_____

_____

_____

_____

_____

_____

_____

_____

_____

Highway 44: What is Homeostasis?

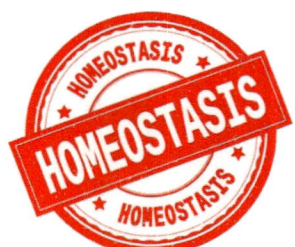

Homeostasis is a state of physical, mental, and emotional stability. This is your ultimate target. Not only have you succeeded with weight loss but now you can triumph with the success associated with long-term weight loss. Your lifestyle changes can become permanent. Your physical anatomy and cognitive clarity will also improve.

Tips to Achieve Homeostasis

1. Eat at Regular Times—Establishing a daily routine for eating times will help you stay organized.
2. Stay positive! Do not let one or two failures stop your forward progress. Remember that this is a journey down a lifetime highway. It is not a quick trip to achieve wellness and homeostasis.
3. Encourage yourself. Some people like to create positive affirmations and say them out loud each day. Some people create a Vision Board. Let your approach to wellness be something personal that becomes part of your life.
4. Reward yourself when you reach certain goals or enabling objectives. Take a short trip. Buy something you've been wanting. Go out with friends. Don't hide out because you aren't in the shape you are working to reach.
5. Eliminate negatives. Reduce or end contact with individuals who may be detrimental to your personal wellness success.

How have you established a homeostasis routine?

_____
_____
_____
_____
_____

Forensic Wellness® Workbook
Your Journey Companion to Wellness

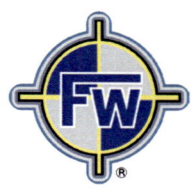

Highway 45: Weight Fluctuation

Remember that your body is a biological machine which is very complex. Optimal throughput for the biological machine is an important factor in losing and maintaining your weight goal.

You are in the weight-loss process for the long haul. Celebrate each pound and ounce of weight loss. However, do not panic if there is an upward fluctuation. Simple things like water retention may be responsible. Figure it out and move on. Don't let it sidetrack you.

What are your identifiers with weight loss fluctuation?

_____

_____

Highway 46: Equilibrium, PAM, and PAW

Losing a pound a month (PAM) sounds slow but over a year that's 12 pounds. Imagine if you could lose two pounds a month. That would be 24 pounds in one year. Weight loss at this pace is sustainable. You are giving your body and mind time to adjust to everything you do and eat.

Losing a pound a week (PAW) would result in you being 52 pounds lighter in one year! This is a realistic goal. It is not some "pie-in-the-sky" dream! It is completely doable with realistic and implementable changes to your lifestyle.

- Say NO to high-calorie soft drinks, desserts or cookies.
- Take a walk and look at the world around you.

When calories consumed and calories burned are equal, then you no longer gain weight. Although this is an easy concept to understand, we humans do not seem to grasp that foundational equation of power in = power out! If you want that extra treat, do enough exercise to burn those calories that same day.

But you are strong enough to take on any challenge ... remember that! You have what it takes to win.

List 5 "Fun Foods" You Enjoy and How Much Exercise and How Long it Will Take to Burn That Many Calories.

_____

_____

Forensic Wellness® Workbook
Your Journey Companion to Wellness

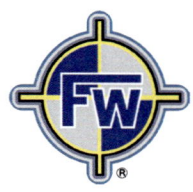

Highway 47: Blood Pressure—Simplified

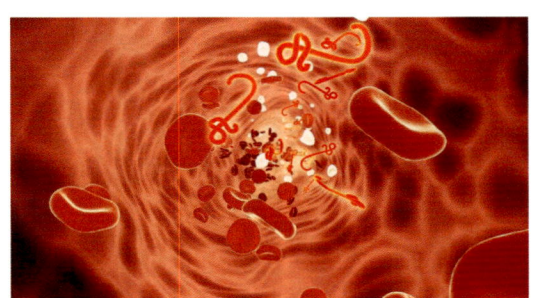

An average adult has 100,000 miles of blood vessels. That's a lot. In fact, it's almost halfway to the Moon or four times around the earth.

For basic math, let's assume a blood pressure reading of 100 over 70 or 100/70 mm Hg.

- 100 mm Hg moves blood through 100,000 miles
- 100 – 70 = 30 mm Hg representing energy added by each heartbeat
- Body requires 30 mm Hg to move blood through 100,000 miles
- High blood pressure due to restricted arteries requires the heart to work harder

Highway 48: Use Your Imagination!

Use your imagination to consider how difficult it would be to build a house or a village, only to have a T-Rex trample everything into the ground. And then be terrorized by a Velociraptor.

Now to your personal weight loss situation. If you want to lose and keep off weight, it's going to require a new attitude about your life in general. You have to realize how important good health is. You must acknowledge that you will have to develop the willpower to say NO! to high-calorie temptations everyday.

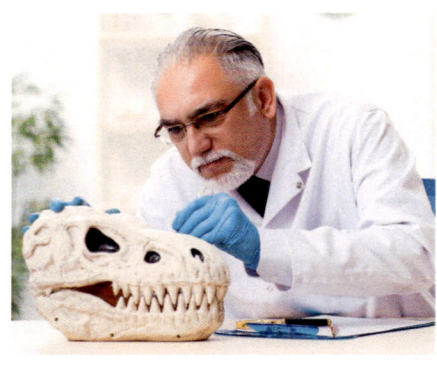

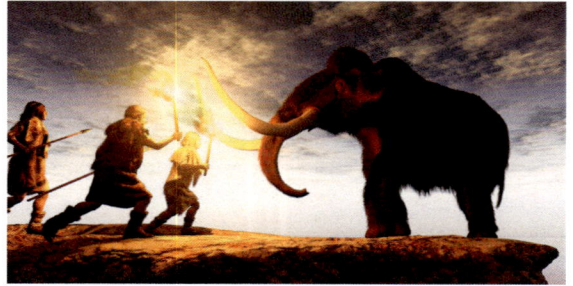

You are evolving. You are realizing that we do not live in a world where daily physical labor is probably required of you. There is no reason to eat all those calories for your occupation. They are simply not required for the type of work you do.

Losing weight is a life-changing decision. Losing weight requires daily action and decision making. Sticking with the decision results in a lifetime of improved health and wellness.

Forensic Wellness® Workbook
Your Journey Companion to Wellness

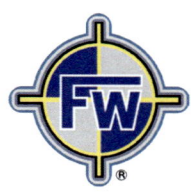

Forensic Wellness® Workbook
Your Journey Companion to Wellness

These decisions and these changes ... they are about much more than weight loss. They are about changing the core fundamentals of personal thought and who you are.

- Are you tired of starting projects, yet never finishing them?
- Are you fed up with not being able to get those really great job opportunities that friends, family, and others may have?
- Are you ready to establish a new and better highway for your life and lifestyle?

You can do this! You have the fortitude deep inside you. Following the *Forensic Wellness*® highway will take you to where you have always wanted to go with your life. The STEM plan establishes a solid foundation for success. You can exercise discipline in your life. You can make good choices. You will become the best version of you.

Your Thoughts:

_____
_____
_____
_____
_____
_____
_____
_____
_____
_____
_____

Forensic Wellness® Workbook
Your Journey Companion to Wellness

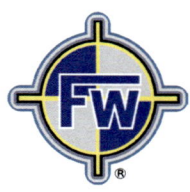

Highway 49: An Explanation of PAM and PAW

Pound A Month—PAM and Pound A Week—PAW are memorable and achievable goals for your weight-loss journey. My actual results are shown in the adjacent Withings Healthmate software graphic. This weight loss may seem like a slow process. It is important remember that if you can master PAM and PAW you will not ever have to go on another diet. You will understand how your body works and how to maintain your target weight.

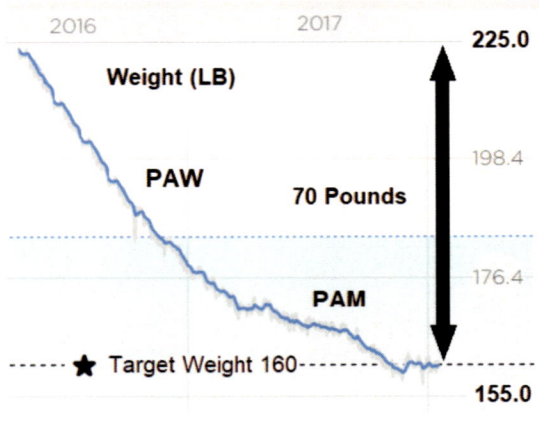

As you are reading this book you can identify many things in your life that take time and effort to accomplish. Life is not easy and achieving objectives requires determination. We must logically assess healthful weight loss over a realistic time frame. Commitment to your health goal can parallel the same diligence and commitment as going to a job each day.

What you eat and how much you eat totals up to a daily calorie count. To lose weight, your daily calorie count has to come down or the daily calories burned must go up.

This workbook does not focus on increasing calories burned. This book focuses on your current lifestyle, eating habits and movement patterns. If you have a very physical lifestyle, then you will be able to eat more. This is easy to accomplish, when you stay with it.

Your *Forensic Wellness*® Lifestyle: It is a numbers formula for Life! Write down the following: Current Weight, Goal Weight, Plan Chosen (PAM or PAW), Date You Can Reach New Goal Weight?

_____

_____

_____

_____

_____

Forensic Wellness® Workbook
Your Journey Companion to Wellness

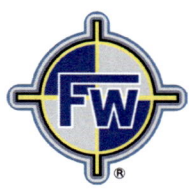

Highway 50: Your Clothing

When you begin to lose weight, your body and physique will change. Your focus, dedication, and decision making has played off. Your clothes are no longer tugging at you when you put them on. Your old clothes are falling off your body.

You have dropped a significant amount of weight and now it's time to buy some new clothes. Let's "walk slow" and think this through before heading off to the clothing store.

Your new clothes represent the new you. Your new clothes communicate your personal image. You have planned for this day. Planning started when you made the commitment to travel the *Forensic Wellness®* highway. Your new clothes will embody your personal self-vision. This is a success moment in life, lifestyle, and health. Enjoy the Process.

Highway 51: Update Your Success Plan

When we look successful, we feel successful. This new girl or guy may have some unique ideas about and contributions for the future. What are your dreams? All journeys begin with one step.

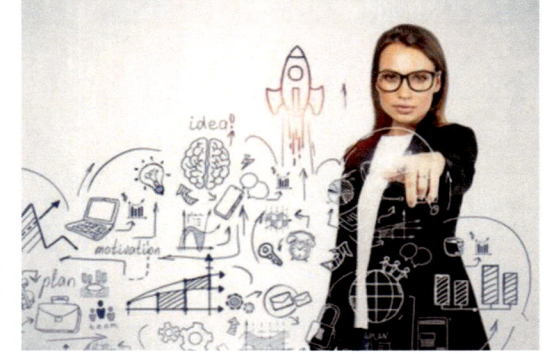

As President Kennedy once said, "Attack your life with all due vigor." Make and put in place calculated decisions about your dreams, goals and plans for the future.

Known, defined, and calculated? Yes. You have reached an important point on the weight loss timeline. Be sure to enter your initial weight, current weight, and time to reach the current weight.

Write down what the new you wants in your life:
_____
_____
_____
_____

Forensic Wellness® Workbook
Your Journey Companion to Wellness

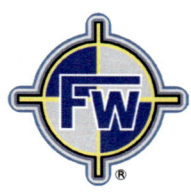

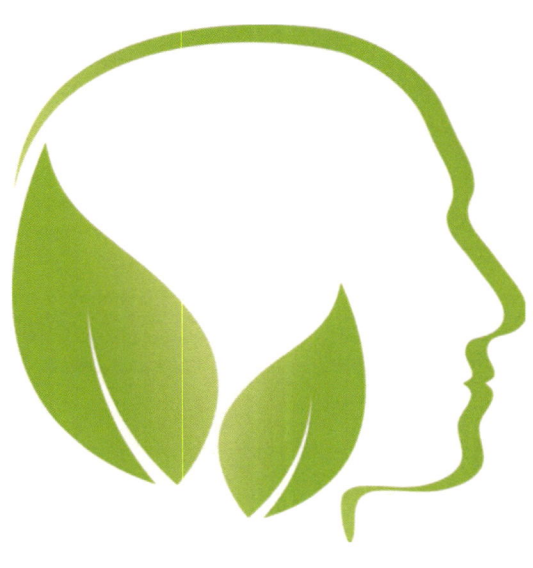

Initial Plateau Time

Initial Plateau Time (IPT) represents how long you and your body took before the weight loss started. If you are using a smart scale to track your weight, the data will document when your weight loss started. The data record will show when your downward sloping trend line began. Up to the point that the trend line is horizontal, representing no change in weight is IPT.

Now you have two lines. IPT is straight and the trend line is the downward slope. If you went to the race track, IPT would be time in the pits and the trend line would be on-the-track or OTT.

As your weight drops, changes will take place in your body. Things will start shaping up. You have more energy now. You have less weight to move with each movement you make. Walking requires less effort. Less weight means less stress on your body. Good physical and mental things are the result of your success.

What are the changes you are experiencing in your new body?

_____
_____
_____
_____
_____
_____
_____
_____
_____
_____

Forensic Wellness® Workbook
Your Journey Companion to Wellness

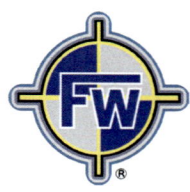

Highway 52: Physique and Lifestyle

Your eating habits are different now compared to when you began the program. Calorie intake is lower and the types of foods you eat are different than when you began the program. You may have enjoyed the 1,000+ calorie hamburger or dessert in the past. That high calorie meal is probably in your rear-view mirror. If your daily calorie maintenance number is 2,000 you have a solid value. The giant hamburger or dessert will blow the daily 2,000 number out of the water.

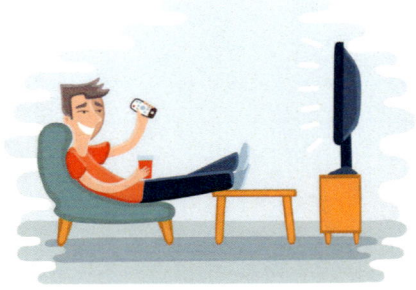

Have you met your goals and do you have future goals?

Calorie splurging and reverting to old eating habits can be disastrous. Bad habits and bad decisions take you in the wrong direction. You have worked too hard to get where you are today. Continue to resist temptation and social pressure. Build up your inner strength and determination!

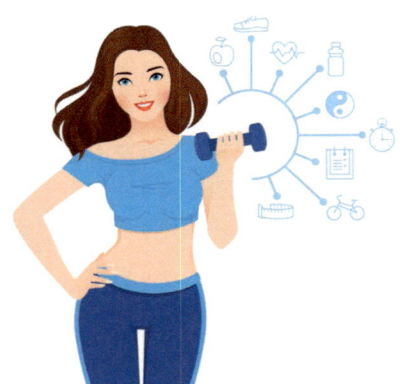

If you feel challenged, then go shopping and try on some new clothes. You have to keep that picture of the new YOU fresh as you transition into this new way of life.

Review your workbook or review your weight loss chart and see how far you've come. Remember the dreams and plans you have been making. If you've created a Vision Board, then studying it each day can help keep you motivated.

Feel great every time you add to your clothing collection. You can take great pride in your accomplishments. Begin to work on your career, education, and personal or entrepreneurial dreams. The further you go down this new pathway of discovery, the easier it will be to stay the course. It is no longer just about weight loss. The overall objective is to creating a better life for yourself and those around you. It's about achieving your dreams. To achieve current and future goals, it requires you to take the first step and keep moving forward.

See how far you have come!

_____

_____

_____

_____

Forensic Wellness® Workbook
Your Journey Companion to Wellness

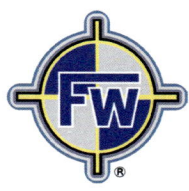

Highway 53: Maintaining an Optimal Physique and Lifestyle

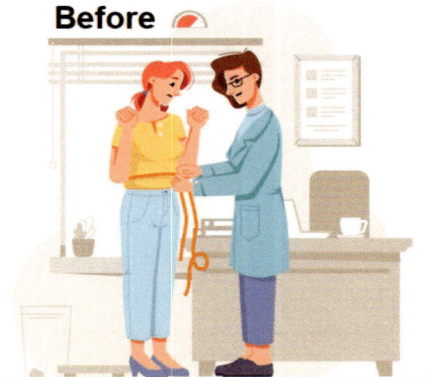

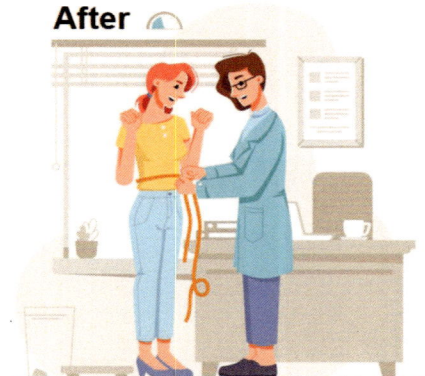

Do you want to remain at your target weight and physique? If the answer is "yes," then it's important to begin creating a new lifestyle that you can enjoy for the rest of your life!

A good way to motivate would be to share your success story with others. All over the world, men, women, and children are struggling with weight and wellness. Processed and engineered foods lead to an overweight body and high-calorie lifestyle. Many people need to hear your story. The more you get out in the world and experience this new version of yourself, the more fun you will have. Your new you will find it much easier to say NO! to high-calorie foods.

You are embarking on a new journey of discovery. How does it feel?

_____

_____

_____

_____

_____

_____

_____

_____

_____

Forensic Wellness® Workbook
Your Journey Companion to Wellness

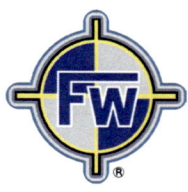

Highway 54: Take Control of Your Health

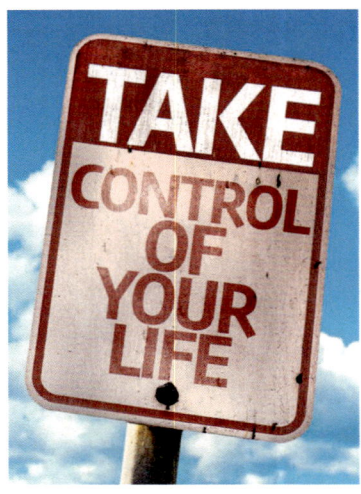

Your health and biomechanical body have changed. There are important benefits of being in good physical shape. Here are success points that you can take pride in accomplishing:

- Decreased body fat
- Increased muscle tone
- Increased physical activity
- Improved mental acuity
- Improved sleep quality

Weight loss reversion is why many weight control plans have not been successful. If you are experiencing or think you may have a problem with reversion get proactive now.

Now is the time to put in place the conscious decision not to revert back to the old lifestyle and weight.

Take action now to control your weight! Remember that the weight you need to lose now is probably a whole lot less than when you first started on the STEM plan. By taking action now, you'll only have to make relatively modest decisions to curb that weight gain. The STEM plan has helped you make huge decisions about what you will eat and how much you eat.

What actions are you taking to control your weight?

_____

_____

_____

_____

_____

_____

Forensic Wellness® Workbook
Your Journey Companion to Wellness

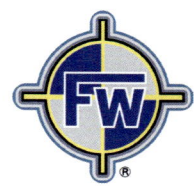

Forensic Wellness® Workbook
Your Journey Companion to Wellness

Highway 55: Progress, Assessment, and Reassessment

Highway 55 is all about your progress on this journey. You've made vast improvements in the way you deal with high-calorie foods. In fact, you've made huge improvements in the way you live life. You're a new person with all new goals. You have a new wardrobe, new ambitions, and you are looking forward to a happy, successful, fun life. Encourage yourself and others who join you on this journey.

Below are a few issues and questions to consider:

- Know your daily calorie count in and out.
- Look at and assess your timeline.
- Was your mental state different at the start of the timeline?
- Has your physical or mental fitness changed from the start of the timeline?
- Do you feel different about weight loss success or failure?

Get Organized and Stay Organized—Life & Lifestyle

Remember to keep recording your progress in your journal. Stay on top of the changes so you can stay in tune with where you are now, where you've been and where you're going. Your wellness and future are opening new doors of opportunity.

Your Life Changes:

_____

_____

_____

_____

_____

_____

Forensic Wellness® Workbook
Your Journey Companion to Wellness

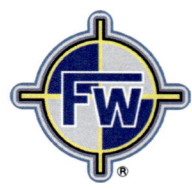

Forensic Wellness® Workbook
Your Journey Companion to Wellness

Highway 56: Do Not Go to the Gym to Lose Weight!

Heading to the gym for a physical workout is good. This can definitely help you achieve a physical workout. Going to the gym and then indulging in a 500-calorie Frappuccino will not help your calorie count.

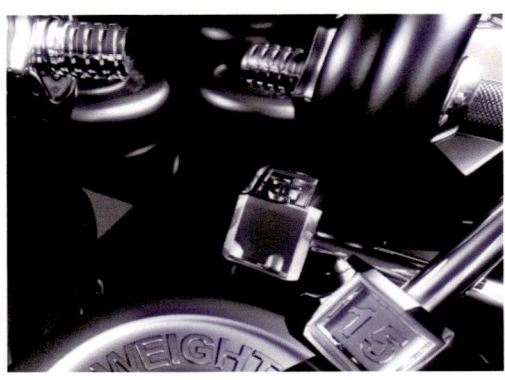

The gym is great place to build up muscle mass and get stronger. You may make some new friends there. But it can give you a false sense of hope when it comes to your eating and weight plan. You may feel like it's okay to eat certain high-calorie foods. Before you know it, you've gained several pounds.

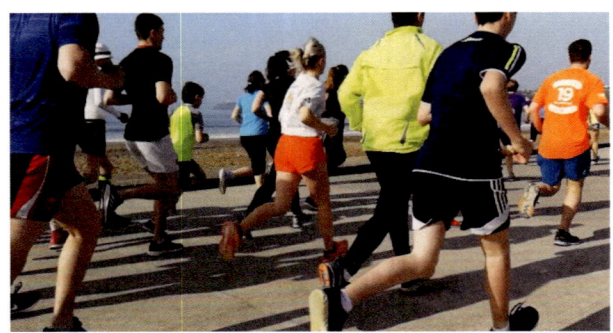

Go for a walk each day. Go for a run. Head to the gym to work out for an hour. But don't get so confident in all those activities that you stop on the way home and eat a big juicy cheeseburger, French fries, and a chocolate shake.

What is your revised weight loss plan? How often does it include exercise ?

_____
_____
_____
_____
_____
_____
_____

Forensic Wellness® Workbook
Your Journey Companion to Wellness

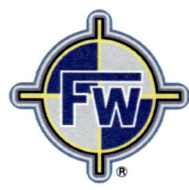

Highway 57: S.T.O.P. is Your Personal Action Plan

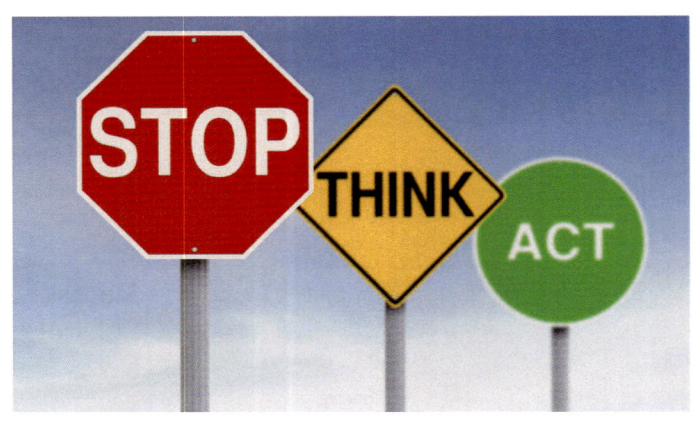

Changing your daily eating activities will change your life. Results are a more healthy, slim, trim, agile, and mentally alert YOU! It is a physical and mental life-day when you look the way you want to in your clothes. You have more physical and mental energy. Your health has improved. You have achieved a major goal on the STEM plan wellness highway.

STOP your body and mind, immediately, on the wellness highway. Stopping gives us an opportunity to clear our mind and focus on our goal. You may have stopped now because of challenges with food selections. This roadblock is a definite learning experience and opportunity.

S is for SIT DOWN. Stop moving and take a break.

T is for THINK. After you've calmed yourself, think about your situation and how you got to this roadblock.

O is for OBSERVE. You need to make comprehensive reality check of your situation.

P is for PLAN. It is only after you have figured out the roadblock issue that you can move forward.

The most difficult part about the **STOP action plan** is to do it. What can serve as a reminder is a STOP sign graphic placed in a visible location. When you see a STOP sign, think about how your life has changed because you are taking control. You are making healthful decisions. You are on the wellness highway.

How and when are you using your personal safety plan?

_____

_____

_____

_____

Forensic Wellness® Workbook
Your Journey Companion to Wellness

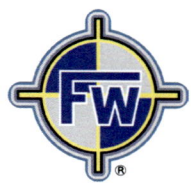

Forensic Wellness® Workbook
Your Journey Companion to Wellness

Highway 58: Tips for Success

The *Forensic Wellness*® STEM plan has permitted you to put in place a healthy reality for your life. You have become more knowledgeable about health and wellness. You are successfully travelling on the wellness highway. Here are some of the topics you have read about and studied in this book:

- Science, technology, engineering, and math = STEM
- Your decision to lose weight and not regain weight
- What you want to eat vs. physique, health, BMR, and BMI
- Understanding is power
- Decision making is power

Remember that this is your mindset against the world of eating everything you want. It involves two important aspects that can make or break you:

- Your craving for high-calorie foods
- Your world: family, friends, media, TV

The food you buy is the food you will eat. Be more aware of what you are eating. Many food products have additives that can have negative effects on your body and hormones. Hormonal imbalances can lead to a roller coaster of mood swings and food cravings.

- Fast-food marketing campaigns
- Processed foods and preservatives
- High-calorie, trans-fat, and sugars
- Restaurant and packaged foods

If you are bored and tempted to eat unhealthy, go for a walk, play a game, call a friend. Developing a healthy quick-response to cravings can be important to wellness. Cravings and temptations are a part of 21st-century life.

What are your food influences and triggers affecting your buying habits?

_____

_____

_____

Forensic Wellness® Workbook
Your Journey Companion to Wellness

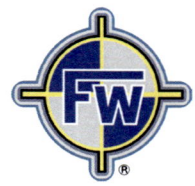

Challenges

Some of the biggest challenges can come from family and friends. We often develop relationships with others based on our personal likes and dislikes. Some elements could include your sense of self and your culture. Social and personal emotional challenges are also factors.

What is your biggest challenge?

_____

_____

_____

Victory Lane

Victory Lane is your destination on the *Forensic Wellness*® STEM plan highway. Lifelong benefits are ahead because you have successfully reached Victory Lane!

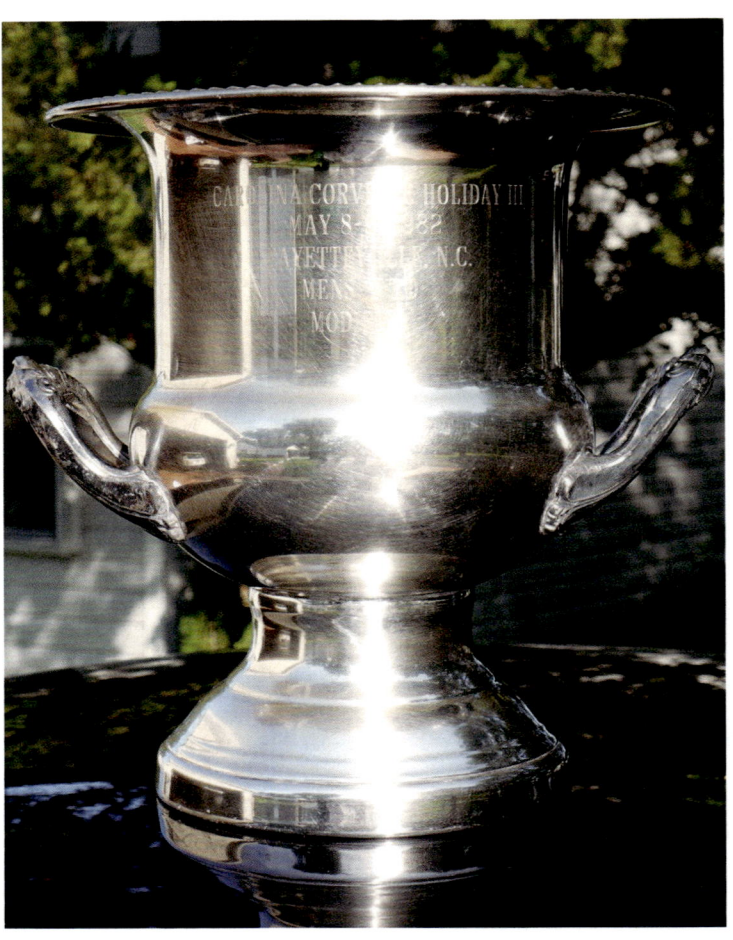

Forensic Wellness® Workbook
Your Journey Companion to Wellness

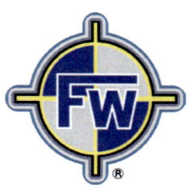

Forensic Wellness® Workbook
Your Journey Companion to Wellness

Highway 59: Choose to Go to the Moon

Why did we choose to go to the Moon? It would be expensive. It would take time. People's lives would be at risk. We did not choose to go to the Moon because it was easy. This was an out-of-this-world objective. Going to the moon served humanity.

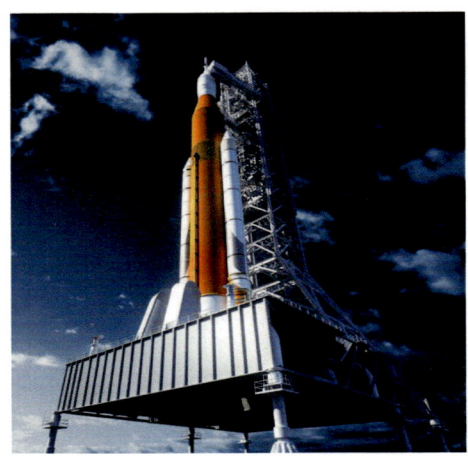

The United States put together some of our best people and most advanced technology. Scientists, engineers and technicians used all their skills and energy. This was a difficult challenge. Mankind, around the world, applauded this success. You have this greatness in your DNA to achieve wellness.

Here is what one of our greatest presidents said:

> "We choose to go to the moon. We choose to go to the moon in this decade and do the other things, not because they are easy, but because they are hard, because that goal will serve to organize and measure the best of our energies and skills, because that challenge is one that we are willing to accept, one we are unwilling to postpone, and one which we intend to win, and the others, too."

—John F. Kennedy, Rice University, September 12, 1962

How high and how far are do you have your sights set? What are your toughest, hardest-to-achieve goals?

_____
_____
_____
_____
_____
_____
_____

Forensic Wellness® Workbook
Your Journey Companion to Wellness

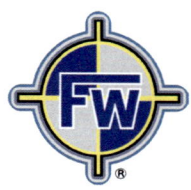

Forensic Wellness® Workbook
Your Journey Companion to Wellness

Highway 60: Your STEM Highway to Wellness

Food and drink are essential fuels for your biologically powered body. Your body, from an energy-in and activity-out analysis, represents a complex biochemical mechanical machine. Simplification of energy-in and activity-out will be scaled down. The right foods and calories-in permit achievement of your optimal weight. Logical lifestyle changes will permit you to maintain your optimal weight for life.

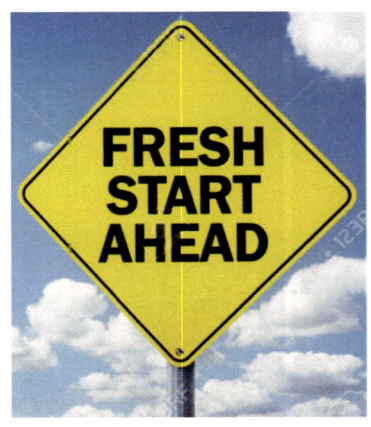

The **Forensic Wellness**® STEM plan is a personally implementable plan. Weight control, weight loss, and countless diet plans are in the news daily.

Forensic Wellness® and the STEM plan is for the 21st century. This contemporary plan brings together daily life elements. Daily life usable STEM elements make weight control successful in the 21st century. To take weight off and keep weight off requires understanding for why people put weight on. Stated another way, if you do not know why you are overweight, then you may not know how to lose weight. If you do not know how to do something it is highly unlikely that you can be successful. When you know where you are going and how to get there you have a high probability for success.

Enjoy your journey on the STEM Highway to Wellness!

Change Your Story, Change Your Life—How Do You Feel Now?

_____
_____
_____
_____
_____
_____
_____

Forensic Wellness® Workbook
Your Journey Companion to Wellness

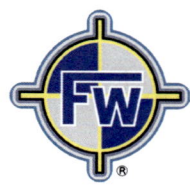

Highway 61: The Winner's Circle—Forensic Wellness® Conclusion

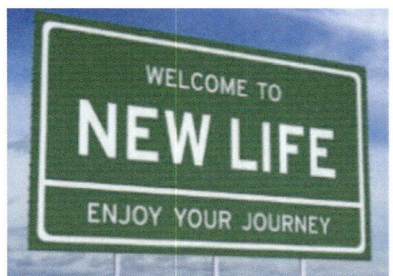

Forensic Wellness is the STEM plan of combining Science, Technology, Engineering, and Math. This is the 21st-century plan to give you a sustainable weight loss and control program. This application of scientific methods creates the program foundation.

The Mediterranean, DASH, and MIND diets are all about healthy foods and healthy eating. The STEM plan takes advantage of the things that work and get rid of what doesn't. You can figure out a personal eating plan that you like. Your plan can be rich in anti-oxidants and emphasizes achieving optimal health.

You have traveled on many highways of ***Forensic Wellness*** to arrive at The Winner's Circle of wellness. You started your journey on one side of the bridge and now you have successfully crossed the bridge.

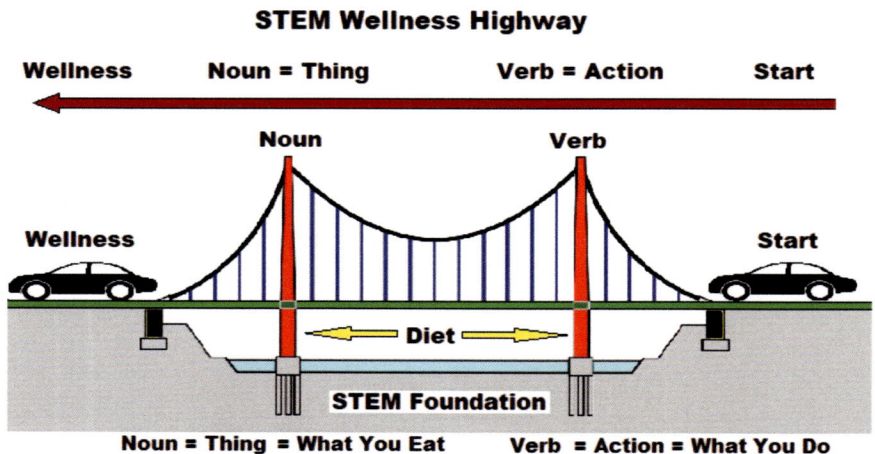

The STEM plan equips you to use your own mind to develop new and healthier relationships with food. We get to the bottom of why you've struggled with weight issues for so long and we find solutions that work. You can get control of your health and your weight and make better choices for a more successful future.

Forensic Wellness® Workbook
Your Journey Companion to Wellness

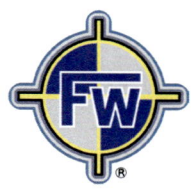

Forensic Wellness® Workbook
Your Journey Companion to Wellness

Highways 62 and 63: Share your STEM Wellness Highway Journey and Visit your destination

We want you to be successful and we believe this plan can work if you will give it a chance. Are you willing to move beyond a failed history of weight gain, calories, food and dieting? If so, you can get your life on a new highway to better health, fitness, and wellness for the 21st century.

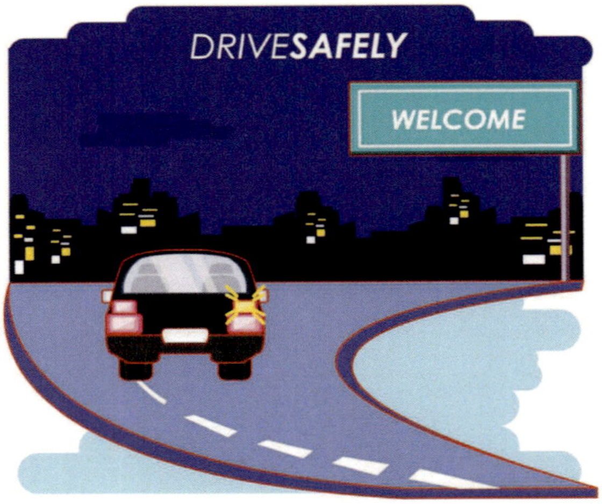

_____

_____

_____

_____

_____

_____

_____

_____

_____

_____

_____

_____

Forensic Wellness® Workbook
Your Journey Companion to Wellness

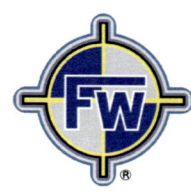

Forensic Wellness® Workbook
Your Journey Companion to Wellness

Highway 64: A New Vision

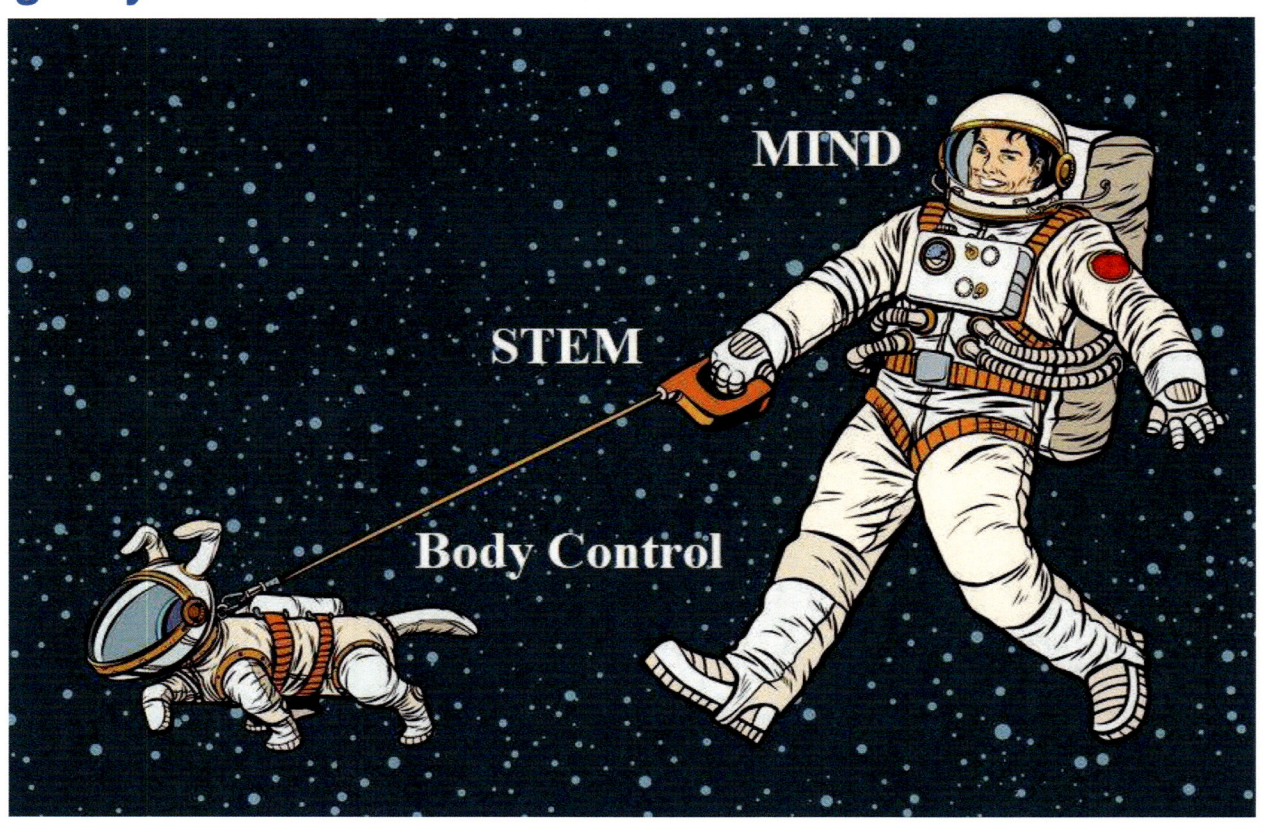

Enjoy your lifelong journey on the STEM highway to better health and wellness.

Final Thoughts:

_____

_____

_____

_____

_____

Forensic Wellness® Workbook
Your Journey Companion to Wellness

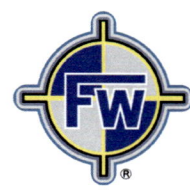

Forensic Wellness® Workbook
Your Journey Companion to Wellness

Forensic Wellness® Workbook
Your Journey Companion to Wellness

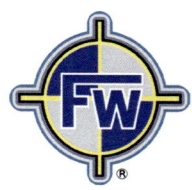

Forensic Wellness® Workbook
Your Journey Companion to Wellness